Redesign your mind
Tools and inspiration for positive mental health

STEFAN MIRAGLIA

Stefan Miraglia © 2019

Stefan Miraglia asserts the moral right to be identified as the author of
'Redesign Your Mind'

Design and typeset by Green Avenue Design

Published by Cilento Publishing, Sydney Australia

ISBN: 978-0-6485587-3-6

All rights reserved. No part of this publication may be reproduced, stored in a retrieval system, or transmitted, in any form or by any means, electronic, mechanical, photocopying, recording or otherwise, without the prior permission of the author or publishers.

The author is not a health care professional or medical professional and the contents of this book are for informational purposes only. Whilst the information and opinions found in this book are written based on information available at the time of writing, and are believed to be accurate according to the best discernment of the author, the content is not intended to be a substitute for professional medical advice, diagnosis, or treatment. Any health concern must be assessed by a doctor. If you think you require assessment, call your doctor or local emergency department immediately. Reliance on any information provided by the author or the contents of this book is solely at your own risk.

wellnessofhealth.com

REDESIGN

Verb

Design (something) again or in a different way.

'Her mind has been redesigned'

Noun

The action or process of redesigning something.

'A positive mindset was achieved thanks to the redesign of his mind'

Synonyms

Remodel, rebuild, remake, upgrade, recondition, revamp, overhaul, modernize, rehabilitate.

YOUR

Determiner

Belonging to or associated with the person that the speaker is addressing.

'Your mind will be redesigned'

Belonging to or associated with any person in general.

'Reading this book will help you on your journey'

Synonyms

His, hers, owned, personal.

MIND

Noun

The element of a person that enables them to think and feel the faculty of consciousness and thought.

'I seek to cultivate positive thoughts for my mind'

A particular way of thinking influenced by a person's profession or environment.

'Her new inspiration drove her to be one of the greatest minds of her time'

Synonyms

Outlook, understanding, reasoning, perception, opinion, attitude, point of view, belief, judgement, feeling, sentiment

5 percent of the author royalties from the sale of this book are donated to mental health organisations of the author's choice. If you would like to nominate an organisation that is doing some good work within the mental health community, please feel free to get in contact.

CONTENTS

PREFACE 9
    A beach story 11
    The fork in the road 13

CHAPTER ONE AN INTRODUCTION TO CHANGE 15
    Why I had to redesign my mind 16
    Merry christmas 22
    Don't forget the chocolates 24
    Footsteps on the beach 25
    Two steps forward, ten steps back 25
    The long road 26
    I call bullshit 27
    The test 30
    Sharing my redesigned mind 31
    The highs and lows 32
    The time machine 33
    The personal trainer for the mind 34
    Feeling good 36
    What do you think? 37
    Am I sad, depressed, or anxious? 38
    Update ready to install 39

CHAPTER TWO HOW SOCIETY HAS SHAPED OUR LIVES 41
    Island of paradise 42
    How society has conditioned our mind 42
    What 'things' are important? 44
    Are you happy? 47
    Post. Like. Share. Repeat. 47
    How many likes did you get? 50
    Entitlement 51
    Knowledge or wisdom 53
    Removing expectations 54

CHAPTER THREE REDEFINING DEPRESSION ... 57
What is de-pression ... 57
Medication and your health ... 60
Change your mindset or change your environment? ... 62
Down but not out ... 64
Help ... 65
Uncle Pete ... 66

CHAPTER FOUR UNDERSTANDING ANXIETY ... 69
Stressed out ... 70
The fear of failure ... 70
Does it really matter? ... 72
My anxiety ... 72

CHAPTER FIVE WHO GIVES A F*CK ... 77
*Redesigning what you give a f*ck about* ... 78
Redesigning yourself ... 79

CHAPTER SIX HOW TO REDESIGN YOUR MIND ... 83
Redesigning your mind ... 85
Steps to redesign your thoughts ... 89
Did I change? ... 90
Redesign your language ... 92
Watch your language ... 93
You should change ... 95
This time next week ... 96

CHAPTER SEVEN GREAT EXPECTATIONS ... 99
Redefining success ... 99
Move the goal posts ... 101
More sex please ... 102
Guilty as charged ... 103

CHAPTER EIGHT THE RIGHT ENVIRONMENT ... 105
Money doesn't grow on trees ... 105
You're only as good as the company you keep ... 107
Cultivate your garden…or find a new one ... 107
God, help me ... 109

Embracing meditation *110*
Using meditation to calm the mind *110*
Using meditation to find your higher self *112*

CHAPTER NINE WHAT CAN I DO TO CHANGE 117
Is it just a placebo? *117*
Practicing yoga *118*
Practicing mindfulness *119*
Redesigning your energy *120*
Count the little wins *123*
Redesigning your diet *123*
Bend like the willow tree *125*
Stay in control, by giving it up *126*
Be average you perfectionist wanker *127*
Write a journal *129*
Breathe *130*
Summarise the day *131*

CHAPTER TEN REDESIGN YOUR PERSPECTIVE 135
Create your own meaning of life *135*
Act as if *136*
Process v outcome *138*

CHAPTER ELEVEN REDESIGNING LIFE 141
Redesign your relationships *141*
Money, money, money *143*
Design your headstone *145*

CHAPTER TWELVE ROADBLOCKS TO YOUR HAPPINESS 147
Oh shit, that didn't work *147*
Finding ways to escape the pain *147*
Redesigning disappointment *148*
Disease *149*
Overwhelm *149*
Waiting to be happy *150*
Talking to everyone about your problems *151*
Locking yourself away *152*

CHAPTER THIRTEEN REDESIGN YOUR LUCK 153
The old man at the fort *153*
Pros and cons *154*
Be a magnet for positive energy *156*
Find your best friend *157*

CHAPTER FOURTEEN YOU CAN CHANGE 159
Redesigning can be challenging *162*
21 Days of change *163*

CHAPTER FIFTEEN A LIFE OF REDESIGN 165
Redesign complete…for now *165*
Shit times will come and go *167*
Where am I now *168*
The mental health stigma *170*
Over to you *172*

THE CHECKLIST TO REDESIGN YOUR MIND 176

STAY IN CONTACT 178

ACKNOWLEDGEMENTS 179

REFERENCES 181

RECOMMENDED READING 182

PREFACE

Have you ever played an active part in the development of your mind? Have you ever worked day and night on cultivating a positive mindset and rationalising any negative thoughts that you may have? For most of us our minds are just made up of what we have learnt from outside influences such as family, friends, school and society. Yes, we have our own beliefs and values but many of the thought processes that we use to decide what makes us happy were not developed by us. There was a time in my life where I realised that I needed to 'redesign my mind'. It was a challenging time but one that I am now grateful for. It was a time where I learnt that my thought processes were largely responsible for how I was feeling. My negative thinking led to anxiety and a deep depression which could only be cured by changing the way I thought. After successfully redesigning my mind, I realised that I had a responsibility to share my successes, my failures and my story with the world – so that you too can find the inspiration to change and grow into the person you deserve to be.

Your 20's are supposed to be your happy years. These are the years where we enjoy life, travel, make mistakes, settle into our career path; and for some it may be where they find love and start a family. My 20's were not always that happy. These years delivered some of the most challenging times of my life. Redesigning my mind was not an easy process, but one that truly helped me understand that many of the problems we have in our lives are a result of our own thinking. I now look at life through a different lens. A lens that searches for the positives in a situation. A lens that no longer envies the success, luck or fortune of another. A lens that no longer fears what can go wrong but instead is optimistic about what could be. A lens that knows I have the tools to push on when times get tough. I feel it is my duty to share my story in the hope of helping you realise that you too can change the way you think. You too can free yourself from the negative thoughts that are the road block to your happiness. You too can level up your mental health. Hopefully my story gives you an inspiring insight into how you can make this happen. Just like any redesign, you are going to need tools. Tools to help you remodel and reshape the way you think and behave. I will give you some of these tools, but it will be up to you to use them. This book is also for me to come back to if I ever lose my way again, as I know that there will be times in life that I will need to dig deeper. You too might need this book to show you the way forward again when times get tough. There will be times in our lives when this book will be our Bible, our shining light to get us through the night. We can't stop the waves, but we can learn to surf. And surfing, riding the emotional waves of life, is exactly what you will be doing by the end of this book. At times you will fall off, which is ok because falling off is just a part of the journey. Falling is how you learn. We do not get depressed because we fall off. We do not get scared of getting up and falling again. We instead use our mind to help us get back on the board and keep moving forward.

After losing interest in the life I was living, I reassessed everything I was doing in order to figure out what it was that I actually wanted in life. I realised that change needed to happen, and the first step was to accept and embrace it. I had to change the way I thought, the way I treated myself, and the way I perceived the world. I know that change isn't easy. To stay in our comfort zone is easy. By accepting that change is good for us and taking action on where we want to be in life, I promise you that great things will happen. This book is for you and me, to inspire us to take action when we know it is much easier to leave things the way they are. This book is written by someone who wants happiness, for someone who wants happiness. Whether you are just looking to find a few more ways to be positive, or you know that you need to totally revamp the way your mind works – this book will have something in it for you. I look forward to travelling the journey with you as you redesign your mind.

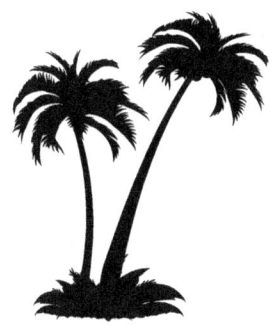

A BEACH STORY

Imagine you are on an island and your friends tell you that there is a beautiful beach on the coast, with water as blue as the sky, pure white sand, secluded and special; however the catch is that to get to the beach you have to walk a treacherous path through the jungle. If you take this path, you know that you are going to have to walk through some shit. There might be parts where you see the coast and stare at it like an oasis. You might start your journey and become jealous of other people who might already be at the beach. You might think that they had it easier than you did. You might question if you are even going the right way. You have never been on this path before, but you push on because you want to get to the beach. You know that this beach is paradise, but you are scared that you will never make it. Your friends might have told you that you are awesome and that someone as good as you would be able to get to the beach with ease. This filled your head with expectations, belief, and maybe the lack of mental preparation for the challenges that you soon faced. *Why is this so hard? I was told that this would be easy.* The constant barrage of shit you have had to go through has really got you down. You fear that the rest of the way is going to be just as bad, and you can't even enjoy the nice parts. Your mind is full of fear and apprehension about what lies ahead and whether you will ever get there or not. You might be full of anxiety, depression or even both.

Eventually you make it to the beach. You can't believe your eyes when you break out of the shrubs and run out on to the sand and into the crystal-clear water. You are exhilarated that you made it. Your mind is full of excitement and joy and you instantly forget about the dark times, the fear, the depression, and those times where you nearly gave up. You are in paradise now and it no longer matters that you faced anxiety and depression to get there.

This story greatly resembles a part of my life. When I was young I was told that my future was going to be great. I was full of enthusiasm, expectation and ready to conquer the world in any way I wanted. Most of my life was going to plan and it wasn't until challenges presented themselves that my emotions took over. Just like in the beach story, my life started with enthusiasm and excitement about getting to paradise. When it wasn't as easy as I thought it would be, anxiety and depression set in. My expectations (which were partly influenced by others) were that everyone who was talented and works hard like I do will get to their beach. We *deserve* our beach. What I didn't know was that nothing is guaranteed, and no one *deserves* anything. But if you were to guarantee anything, it would be that challenges will present themselves along the way. Just like the journey to the beach, my life went through some tough times that eventually led to something special. The upcoming journey to redesign my mind was one that would change my life forever.

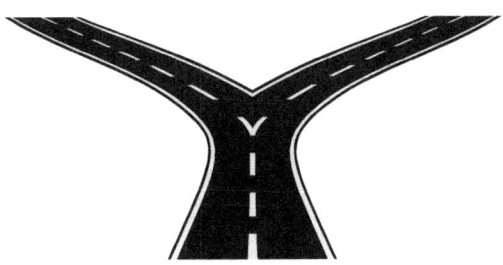

THE FORK IN THE ROAD

There is a fork in the road… Do you take the left track (lots of money but less time to enjoy it); or do you take the right track (minimal money but a happy life)? Challenging choice isn't it? We know that most of us set up our lives to chase the left track – which we think is right but may actually be wrong. Maybe you can make your own track? For most of my early life I was set on the left track with goals focused on looking into the horizon – often losing touch with the present. We are all lured by the thought of money, expensive toys, houses and everything else. But is this really what makes us happy or is this just what society has taught us? You may have been questioning your path before starting this book. Only you can figure out whether you are on the right path or not – however what this book will show you is that it is okay to not be on the right path. It is okay to turn around, go left, right, up or down, or even just stay where you are. You might have some parts of yourself that you truly never want to change, and that's ok. I eventually found that my existing path was not for me – and after a great deal of anxiety and depression, I decided to redesign my mind. Sometimes the problem is that our vision is so clouded with our own bullshit that we can't see that we are going the wrong way. You don't have to be angry, sad, depressed, jealous, anxious, tense, stressed or disappointed any longer than you choose to be. You can start being the happy, grateful, unique, appreciative, thankful, carefree, easy-going, free-flowing, fun, person you want to be.

At this stage you are probably questioning how this is going to happen. That's great! It means that you really want to change. It is time for you to release yourself of any excuses that are stopping you from being the person you want to be. Hey, I'm not saying that I have morphed into a super-human perfect being, but what I can say is that I feel a lot better about myself and have the tools to deal with what goes wrong in life. This book is designed to bring you thought-provoking inspiration, laughter, tools to cultivate a positive mindset and a belief that you can change too. I urge you to do as I have done and throw yourself into the journey of redesigning your mind. Start by accepting yourself for who you are today and committing to working on who you want to be tomorrow.

CHAPTER ONE
AN INTRODUCTION TO CHANGE

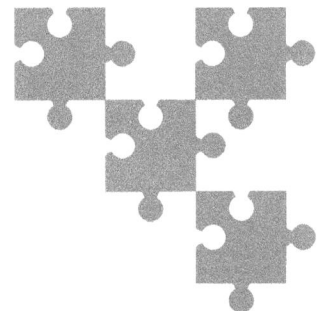

I am not a psychologist but what I do have is a life experience that may be similar to yours. I have lived a life of great expectations and found that the challenges of life have sometimes been too great to bear – all because of my thoughts on how things *should* be. My story is not one of someone who won a gold medal in the face of adversity – my story is of the average person who put themselves through emotions of anxiety and depression unnecessarily and made the decision to change. You are not alone. There are many people going through challenges day to day that you are not even aware of. Many of the tools that I will go through are not new to the world, but they will help you relate to what you may have previously heard on a deeper level. After seeing how I used these tools and techniques in my story, you too can redesign how you think. Since starting my mental health blog, wellnessofhealth.com, many people have come to me to share their fears and challenges. Mental health is silent. Most of the time we have no clue that someone may be struggling. You know that friend that you may be envious of, who seems to have the perfect life? Well they might actually be doing it tough – but you wouldn't know because they hide their emotions and you only see their facade. When I went through my challenges with anxiety and depression, many of the people that knew me couldn't believe it. They thought that my life was relatively easy and that I was confident, charismatic, fun and happy. As I share my story you will understand that at the time, this couldn't have been further from the truth.

In 2008 three million Australians were living with anxiety and depression (Beyondblue.org.au, 2019); we live in 'the lucky country', yet more than 1 in 10 people are living with these challenges. This was over ten years ago, and I shiver at the thought of how bad things are now. It is not just Australians who are facing mental health issues. In the USA, 12.7% of people aged 12 and over have recently taken anti-depressants (Cdc.gov, 2017). The whole world needs to start thinking about mental health and how we can make things better. I even wonder how many people have had mental health issues but aren't even aware of it. Or even how many people have mental health issues but choose to do nothing about it. Whatever the number, it is important to remember that we are not the only ones struggling with mental health, and not the only ones who will benefit from redesigning our minds. It is hard to comprehend that there is a community of people dealing with mental health issues, but because of the mental health stigma we are often afraid to talk about it and help each other. It is time to raise the awareness that it *is ok not to be ok*, and that there is nothing wrong with talking about it.

Just like life, you might think that some parts of this book are going to suck, but there will also be times where you say that this is awesome. I know that I really would have appreciated this book being given to me at any stage of my life, so I hope you can too. I am not here to motivate you or to get you to do anything you don't want to do. I am here to inspire you, because if I can find inspiration at the bottom of the barrel, you can too.

WHY I HAD TO REDESIGN MY MIND

I am your average 30-year-old guy from Adelaide, Australia, who never thought that he would be writing a book about facing mental health challenges. Being someone that is ambitious, confident and enjoys having a laugh – I just thought anxiety or depression would never happen to me. My heritage is Italian, and my family has instilled the traditions and values of family, hard work, and being the best person, you can be. I was a bit of a brat as a child but as I grew older I matured into a hard-working young man with integrity and respect, a man who loved the idea of shooting for the stars. School was easy, I had lots of friends, a girlfriend, was pretty popular and I didn't even have to try to obtain academic success. I aced Uni too without having to try. Then I landed a graduate position (I was the first pick of over 2,000 people that applied for the role) and started working for one of Australia's largest banks. I flew up the ranks pretty quickly and by 23 I was managing a business lending portfolio of over $80 million. It was a time when anxiety became part of my life. Anxiety left me feeling scared that I wasn't actually skilled at my work and instead had just talked others into promoting me into my position. I was scared that I would be exposed as a fraud and not actually worthy of success.

I bought my first house at age 21 and felt like I was on the right track to achieving being 'rich' by 30, owning a Ferrari with lots of money. All of my mates would come over to hang out at my house, throw parties and just have a great time – all under my roof. I was confident, arrogant, cocky, and felt as if things were going to keep going up and up for me. My work colleagues would tell me how lucky I was. I remember thinking about how lazy and unmotivated they were. I wondered why they felt a need to see everything as too hard. I was in a conflict with myself as part of me was confident and wanted to strive for success, and part of me was plagued with anxiety. Every decision I made turned out to be a good one and it seemed like I really did know it all. Although anxiety was at the back of my mind, I seemed to be on the right path, ready to continue to 'cruise' through life. Hah! What a Jackass. Now instead here I am at 30, with no Ferrari, writing a book about cultivating happiness. Wow things really do change!

At 23 I planned a holiday to the USA with my brother and two of my best mates. Whilst I had travelled previously, this was destined to be the trip of a lifetime. I remember thinking that I would go away for the holiday of my life and then when I got back I would search for a wife and be married sometime around 25 or 26 (yeah sure). This trip was something I had looked forward to all my life. It meant so much to me and came with the added pressure that I wanted it to be an experience that my brother, mates and I would see as the time of our lives. I look back now and see that the anticipation and expectation I put onto this trip was unrealistic and sure to bring about negative emotions.

I was on the plane just about to land in Hawaii on route to New York City, when I felt an instant wave of sickness. To this day I am not sure if it was the descent of the airplane, the chicken dinner served on the plane or the anxiety of the anticipation that I was about to go on this life changing holiday that caused me to feel sick. Whatever the cause, anxiety was what followed. I was so vain that I became anxious that I was going to be sick and throw up my last meal of protein –which would mean that my muscles would shrink by the time I got off the plane. I was also anxious that all of a sudden, this holiday may not turn out as expected. This attack was different to any form of anxiety I had ever felt back at home. A switch had been flicked that had changed me from the coolest person around to an anxious shaking nervous mess. If I was back home I would have thrown up everywhere, taken the day off work and started again the next day. But not here. Not at this exact moment. The pressure of making this holiday the time of our lives created an anxiety that I didn't understand at the time. What would all the boys say if I came back and told them that I didn't have any good stories, or pick up any girls while I was on holiday? Not all of these thoughts were at the front of my mind, but I know they were stored somewhere in the back. Whether the switch was flicked by the airplane food or not, something changed inside of me and I was instantly a different person. I became scared that I wouldn't be able to eat my next meal. Scared of ruining the holiday. Scared of being a loser. *I never get sick*. Maybe something *is* wrong. Maybe I need a doctor? *Why now?*

Maybe if I had thrown up, the anxiety would have been released with the hurl of spew that would have flown across the aisle. But instead I held it inside. I tried to keep my pain from anyone else and hoped that it would go away. This is exactly how I and a lot of other people hold their emotions. We suppress our emotions. We send it to our gut, to our head, or our back or our neck. And pain, sickness and disease start. I had fallen into a spell of anxiety and depression.

For the next few days I was extremely sick, struggling to keep any food down. I created my own General Anxiety Disorder (GAD), which is basically feeling anxious about feeling anxious. I was so anxious that I was going to be sick that I instantly lost all of my confidence. I went from being the coolest bloke that everyone looked up to and became an insecure, introverted, anxious, delusional, disengaged person. This wasn't who I am. *Everyone in the USA is going to think I'm a loser. Why now? Why can't I just feel better and have a laugh?* The pressure became so large that all I wanted to do was go home. I wanted to be home and safe in my little bed, with mum and dad there to comfort me and tell me that it was all going to be ok. Throughout the holiday I had a few fun moments, but the fear of the fear was too much to truly be free and enjoy myself, resulting in depression. *Why am I feeling like this? I am on holiday with my bro and two best mates; I should be having the time of my life. What's wrong with me? I must be sick; it's a stomach bug from the plane.* I was so disorientated at times that I didn't know which way I was going. Somehow, I managed to at least *look like* I was holding it together and a few girls even tried to pick me up. But I pushed them away for one reason or another. I was hopeless. Who knows what my brother and best mates were thinking. To make things worse, I felt like I had let everyone down, including myself. As the holiday came to an end I enjoyed a few good times, but they were nothing special. Maybe it was a slight release of pressure because I didn't have to impress anyone as much anymore and most of the damage was already done. I could finally go home and get back on with my life and never have to go on holiday again. At least it was over now. Or so I thought…

Unfortunately coming back home-made things worse because everyone wanted to know how much fun I had while on my holiday. Friends and work colleagues were looking forward to hearing all about my stories. Usually I would engage in storytelling and enjoy banter with the gang, but when I got home I realised that this was now the old me. Unfortunately, the stories I told weren't that great and the touring party's main memories involved laughing at me because I was in such a daze and not myself throughout the trip. I thought the cause may have been the food poisoning which was still lingering in my body some five weeks after that dispiriting getaway. Before leaving for the USA I loved travel, but this disastrous holiday made me think that travel sucked, and I didn't want to leave my little bubble at home.

Something was happening to me and there was no logical explanation as to why I felt this way – other than the 'stomach bug'. Work suffered, personal life suffered, my friendships suffered, my love life suffered, and I felt alone. I went to the doctor's and explained my symptoms. After running a few tests he explained that it was a mild case of anxiety. I laughed it off. *'Me? Anxiety? No way; you're wrong it's a stomach bug, but I'll get over it'*. I dismissed a doctor who had probably been practicing for 20 years as if he was a mate at a BBQ talking shit about something he knew nothing about. I then sought to draw my own conclusions, thinking maybe it was the pressure of my job *(yes, that's it Stef. It's your job; the workload is too much and it's your job; not you, you're fine it's your job that makes you anxious…)* and eventually I asked to step down from my high flyer management role; however, my boss told me to stick it out because I was good at what I did. With his guidance I did stick it out and I continued to push through.

At the time one of the most challenging parts was that everyone knew me as an outgoing, fun, confident, charismatic, energetic, open and cheeky person. So when I got back from the USA, everyone expected that to continue but it didn't. I had changed. I remember taking a girl on a dinner date and when I looked at the menu everything made me feel sick. I ordered something but ate practically none of it, using the excuse that I had eaten before and that's why I wasn't hungry. Anxiety had officially taken over, but I was still in denial.

I don't know what or how it happened, but by some sheer miracle I woke up one day and the constant brain fog was gone, and things had gone back to normal. I just felt a little less shit and then before I knew it I was happy again. Everyone must have noticed because one of my mates even said how it was 'good to have you back Stef; you were in a bit of a low for a while'. I remember thinking wow that was a weird part of my life.

I was now back on top of the world and couldn't believe that I was recently so deranged. Life was so good that my confidence soared to a new high. It felt like the serotonin and endorphins that my body released were now flooding back to the parts of my brain that had been blocked and unused for so long. When this new rush of serotonin and endorphins are released, your happiness is at a new high and you may develop a sense of overconfidence. Well my confidence soared, and I felt like I deserved to hit new highs.

At the same time I could see that some of my mates were now starting to enjoy their own successes which made me question what I was going to do next with my life. I felt I was not progressing fast enough in my banking job. One book that I now wish I had read at this time was *Thinking, Fast and Slow* (2011) by Daniel Kahneman. Daniel talks about a term 'regression to the mean' which blew my mind when I read it. 'Regression to the mean' is basically how anything (people, sports teams, winning streaks) will eventually return to the mean. For example, if a company is outperforming the market in sales, eventually it will lose sales to other competitors as they will regress in some way and the lesser companies will improve. I have been an *overachiever* all my life, always doing better than the average. It was eventually going to happen that some of my peers would catch up and even do better than me. My mindset was that because I was good in the past, I would be great in the future – which was totally wrong. I wanted to find a way to stay above the mean when instead I *should* have been bracing myself for the upcoming regression to the mean.

Money was a key driver of mine. I thought about how I could make more money and decided to start my own business. Whilst working full time, I completed two diplomas and set up two companies. Now for anyone that has started in business before, you know how it is; many late nights, lessons, and a great deal of uncertainty. Coming from a job with a guaranteed income and certainty of what I was doing day in day out, this was a challenge. With my overconfidence I totally underestimated how hard this would be and stepped into the world of business at the age of 25. Now keep in mind that after returning from the USA holiday and getting better, things were only back to normal for a short time before I decided to overload myself with work. It was a big load to take but I knew that I just had to get it done and that once I started my business, life would be 'much easier'. Oh yeah, and I forgot to mention that by now I owned two investment properties with two sets of mortgages to repay. This was the extra financial burden which increased the pressure to be financially successful. My last day at the bank was much harder than I thought and it was tough to say goodbye. My last work drinks were a great party. When I left it felt like I was standing on the outside of a family home looking in at a family enjoying their Christmas dinner – even though I chose to leave that family. Thoughts of regret, uncertainty, and excitement were all rushing around my mind.

Monday. Day one and the overwhelming feeling came on pretty quickly. Two weeks into my business I was back at the doctor's; with tingling hands, heart palpitations and more. The doctor gave me the same old story about anxiety and I agreed. *I agree this time; you know what I've just started a new business so I am a little stressed and the doctor is right. Stef you need to relax a bit.*

But I didn't relax. I was working seven days a week, having no time for family and friends, and even when I was with them I was thinking about work, or trying not to spend money because I wasn't sure if I had any income that week. I lost my presence and quickly became neurotic and pensive. I started worrying about the worrying, and I couldn't escape it. One night I went out with the boys to try and escape and I got drunk, really drunk. A few days later I woke up to a weird feeling which felt like a tension headache. I've never had a headache in my life. It felt kind of like the time in the US when I was in a daze; but this was much worse because I couldn't think straight. I was cloudy, almost spinning. I remember that I wanted to spend the day in bed and relax, but I pushed on and went to work because I couldn't afford to lose momentum. I remember meeting with clients and it felt as if I was drunk. Clients knew nothing different – well I think so anyway because they still did business with me, but I was struggling. The pressure was huge as my body and mind were both tense. I went back to the doctor's fearing the worst *(Oh what a coincidence Stef, now that you have started your own business and have no sick pay or backup from the bank, you've caught an illness – it's not 'just' anxiety anymore).* This mind fog, dizziness, instability or whatever you want to call it – took over my life.

I underwent numerous doctors' appointments and tests including an MRI on my head (too bad they didn't find the stubbornness of my brain) and eventually a kind doctor said, 'Stef, you are putting yourself under a lot of pressure at the moment, and you're struggling with the fear of the unknown. It is time for you to take some medication to help you relax.' He prescribed me anti-depressants which could have relieved my anxiety. Of course, I was too stubborn to take them. I promised myself that I would relax more. For the next two years I ignored the stress; I ignored my body and I suppressed my emotions even further. I ignored the consistent 'mind fog' or 'disassociation' where my mind was in a constant state of hypertension caused by stress. I would wake up feeling fine but moments later the daze would return. I was sure it would all go away once my business picked up and things became better. The business did pick up, and things were going pretty well. Yes, I was working long hours, but it was ok. The mind fog was still there but to be honest I actually forgot what it felt like to live without it. I just accepted it and continued to push through the stress. I couldn't leave to go overseas on any holidays because who would run the business while I was away? I didn't care about going overseas anymore anyway because I would just get sick like the last time. *Travel sucks*. When I met with friends or family, instead of the conversations revolving around fun times, last night's football game, going out, swapping funny stories or having a laugh it just revolved around my business. There was no refuge from this feeling of being locked into uncertainty and anxiety no matter where I was. Maybe you can relate? Maybe there is something in your life that has taken over your identity and defines who you are?

MERRY CHRISTMAS

It was Christmas holidays and my friends went on a road trip to a holiday house – which I couldn't go 'in case something happened with the business'. After 18 months of suppressing my emotions, the sustained pressure became too much, and I let it all out to my dad. I cried on my parents couch while he consoled me, noting that he had no idea that I felt this way. I put the reasons of anxiety and depression down to the pressure in my head – and not the other way around. I still blamed some disease or something wrong with me, because it couldn't be stress or anxiety that was doing it. I thought it could be my eyes, my neck, my back, my diet, anything except for my mind. Dad stood by me on my wild goose chase of potential diseases other than anxiety. I also blamed the doctors that I'd seen 18 months ago saying that they hadn't done all the required tests and *should* have done more to find the real disease. I went back to more doctors, chiropractors, physios, eye specialists, ENT's, neurologists, and had numerous scans, which all led to the same definitive conclusion. Anxiety. I used Google to try and self-diagnose which produced numerous potential diseases that my symptoms could be caused by. Anxiety was on the list but I ruled it out because I was only anxious due to this mysterious disease. *Yeah, good one Stef.* My moment of acceptance only came after an appointment with a renowned neurologist that my family had pulled a few strings for me to see. Within minutes of my appointment, she confirmed my ailment. She had seen it before. She knew it well. I was scared and then disappointed when she confirmed that my diagnosis was anxiety and anxiety alone.

Embarrassed and ashamed, I finally accepted that it was anxiety, but I didn't really want to do anything about it, and I definitely didn't want to take the anti-depressants prescribed. Dad finally put his foot down and said that it was all in my head – and that it was up to me to decide whether to take the medication or not; but given that a renowned neurologist confirmed that the medication would help, Dad thought I should take it. But I refused to take the medication and Dad was not happy with me that day! I was still a little baffled that anxiety could cause me to be in a daze 24-7, to stop me from thinking clearly, to cause pressure in my head and neck, and to make my body tense. Accepting that I had anxiety was like accepting defeat, as if I was weak, and there was no longer any excuse for feeling this way. This led me to anxiety's best friend, depression. I now blamed the business as the reason for my anxiety, when in fact it was just the trigger. Thoughts ran through my mind; *Why couldn't I handle this? The business seemed like something I was going to do really well at, why has it stressed me out? Why am I such a loser now, when I was the king only a few years ago? I could stop the business but what do I do next? What would everyone think if I stopped this business? Who am I anyway? I am weak. What am I doing?*

I remember hearing stories of other people's success which made it hurt even more. The regression to the mean was now happening and boy was I regressing. I had wasted so much time, money, effort, blood, sweat and tears on a business that I now considered a failure. My perfect record at making life decisions was now over – and I couldn't handle it. I couldn't handle the fact that I had failed at something. I couldn't handle that I couldn't handle the stress. Depression now set in.

A deep depression lasted a few months – but each day with depression feels like a life sentence. Being self-employed definitely made it worse because this time I didn't have a boss to help me get through it. Instead I was able to spend most of my time at home and started to withdraw from friends and family. I soon decided that it was time to sell my business and start something new. I wrongfully blamed the business for a lot of my stress, anxiety and depression. One of the hardest things I did at the time was to announce to everyone that I was selling my business and I didn't have any positive news or announcement of what was next. This was the first time in my life that I had no idea of my next step. I lost all meaning as I didn't know who or what I was anymore.

DON'T FORGET THE CHOCOLATES

Being in such a depressed state makes you incapable of making any decisions, especially life altering ones. Something as simple as going to the shop and choosing what type of chocolates you want to take to a friend's house was impossible. It's funny to look back on now, but I remember going to a friend's house for dinner one night and popping into the shops to grab some chocolates. I spent 15 minutes standing there trying to decide. *M&M Peanut are on sale in a 500-gram box, but he doesn't like M&M Peanut so I'm not sure. What about a bag of Snickers Mini? They look okay but you only get a few bars in a pack so I don't know if there's much value there. Ok, that's it, I am getting a box of Maltesers *walks 10 steps from the chocolate aisle*. You know what, I better not get the Maltesers because I don't really like them and I want something we can all share. Hmm how much sugar is in this block of chocolate? Oh, wow, that's ridiculous. Wow, there's a new flavour Cookies and Cream, ok I am definitely getting that. But they are on sale as 2 for 1, so I have to choose another block to go with it. Or do I just get two Cookies and Cream? No that would be silly, get something different to try…*

I am sure that some of you might be laughing with me on this one; but the unfortunate fact is that this is caused by a total lack of confidence and full insecurity in the present moment. It was also inevitable that I naturally changed my mind about 50 times about closing the business. I would send in a job application only to email them the next day and say that I no longer wanted to apply; only to call them a few days after my email, asking if I could put my application back in. The chocolates weren't the only thing I had trouble deciding on! The fact that I wanted to be a financial planner when I was younger came to the forefront of my mind. I loved investing and wanted to help people with money, so I decided to enrol in a financial planning course. I saw this as a positive step forward, but I was frozen by the fear of making another wrong decision. I emailed them and cancelled my enrolment. Only to email them again saying I wanted to re-enrol; only to email again saying cancel; and then eventually saying enrol. I still have the email chain with about 10 emails of me changing my mind. I can laugh now, but at the time it wasn't funny, and I know that some of you have faced the same challenge. I had a complete fear of making the wrong decision – chocolates or not.

FOOTSTEPS ON THE BEACH

One afternoon my dad took me for a walk which resulted in the moment that I knew how far I had fallen. Not only was I dragging myself through the mud, but I was taking my whole family with me. Dad suggested I finally try the anti-depressant medication that my doctor prescribed. Whilst I had thoughts of suicide as a way out, it wasn't really what I wanted. I wanted the pain to end, and dying would be an easy option, but luckily, I concluded that I didn't want to take my own life; I just wanted to be happy again. I told myself that no matter how bad things were now, even if I just had one day of pure happiness, one moment of pure laughter, it would all be worth it. My goal became to be happy again. I know that at the time it is not easy, but we have to understand that any dark thoughts are just thoughts; just like how you might think 'I want to slap this person', or 'I would love to walk out of here' on a bad day at work. You don't have to act on these thoughts at all and you don't have to criticise yourself for having these thoughts. So please understand that depression is not a life sentence. We will work on healing these wounds later on as we travel our journey of change.

TWO STEPS FORWARD, TEN STEPS BACK

So I established that I didn't want to kill myself, I just wanted to be happy (just like finding that paradise beach I talked about earlier). I finally agreed with my dad and decided to take the anti-depressants. They say that anti-depressants make you worse before you get better; and what made it worse was my thoughts of self-defeat – the waving of the white flag, having to take a drug to make me feel good. As someone who had lived a relatively drug free life, who didn't even take Panadol, it made it tough. On the third day, dark thoughts were running through my mind and I fell to a new low. The next morning I made the first true decision I had made in the last three months. This was the first time I stood up for myself. This was the first time that I accepted the challenges ahead of me and blamed only myself for my past. I accepted that I had put myself through anxiety and depression and that I was going to do whatever it took to feel happy again without having to take medication. I then walked out of my room, threw out the anti-depressants and said *'Dad, I am not taking this stuff anymore. I know it has only been 3 days, but I am going to start this journey by myself. I am going to do everything within my power to get better, and then when I have tried everything, if I am still feeling shit I will take the meds. But I promise you that I am going to try and do this without medication, and it all starts right now.'*

I could see that my dad was concerned that I was giving up on the medication so soon. He only wanted the best for me, and he believed that we should listen to the doctors and stop avoiding the medication. But I had made up my mind. I knew that the road would be long, but one that I had to take. I know that it is not easy if you are in this state. I know that you have to prove to everyone that you are not crazy and that you are actually getting better. I know that most importantly you have to prove it to yourself that you can get through this and you can be happy again. That day when I decided to move forward, where I decided to accept my actions instead of blaming something else, when I decided to take my life back into my own hands, was the day that led to me changing my life.

THE LONG ROAD

They say that the man who moves mountains starts by moving the smallest stone. And for me I really did start by moving the smallest stone. I stopped Googling what might be wrong with me and accepted that I was anxious and depressed, and moved into what I could do to improve my situation. I will talk more about what I did to redesign my life later on, but for now I want you to know that this is how you start your journey. You start by taking one small step. There is no point looking up at the mountain in front of you, it is all about looking at the first step. Maybe your story is 'worse' or 'not as bad' as mine. Whichever of the two it doesn't matter – but I know that there are many people out there who have had smaller challenges and unfortunately decided that the only way out is by taking their own life. They are the motivation behind this book. It doesn't matter if your story is easier or harder than mine or anyone else's. What matters is what you do next to redesign your life. Do you want to accept that your story and challenges are harder than anyone else's and do nothing? Or do you want to accept this challenge in the hope of a better life? These are questions that only you can answer. Whilst I didn't end up using anti-depressant medication (after day 3), I want you to know that it is totally fine to use medication (remember 13% of US adults are with you too). There is no magic solution. What works for some will not work for others and vice versa. The tools in this book will help regardless of your choice. That said, I believe the only way to increase your happiness in the long term is by changing the way you think and changing the way you live. Now is the best time to start making the changes and no one else can make them but you. You may have all the tools and all the help in the world – but a clear mind and happiness can be created by you and only you. I had awesome friends and family behind me. I had all the support I needed, and really there was nothing too wrong with my life on the surface other than the fact that I had a business that was stressful – however my life was a shambles because of my mindset. It was not until I decided that I was going to take charge of my life that things started to change. Everyone can love you and help you as much as they want, but until you get up from rock bottom and stand up on your own two feet, nothing will change. You might have the most supportive partner, or you might be the most supportive partner and not understand why you can't fix someone. I can tell you straight up that no one can 'fix' anyone. People can only 'fix' themselves. You can help them yes, and you can guide them, but know that you can lead a horse to water, but you cannot make it drink. In this book I share with you what I did to stand on my own two feet and how you too can change your life.

I CALL BULLSHIT

For anyone who has watched *The Wolf of Wall Street*, there is a quote from Jordan Belfort that I think we can all relate to. 'The only thing standing between you and your goal is the bullshit story you keep telling yourself as to why you can't achieve it.' Is this you? I know that I am guilty of telling myself bullshit in the past. How many stories have you made up to make yourself feel better? Things like 'I'm too busy at the moment' or 'no one understands how hard it is for me' or 'I'm waiting for the right time'. These are all bullshit excuses. I only know that they are bullshit excuses because I am a bullshit artist myself (only on the odd occasion these days). I had all the excuses in the world when I was at my lowest point. 'Oh, it must be an illness' and 'I'm not anxious, this is just all caused by the stress of my business' and 'I only feel this anxious and depressed because of my headache and dizziness' (*no Stef, you actually have a headache and dizziness because of your anxiety and depression!*). Even when I wasn't anxious or depressed, I would still make excuses when something seemed too hard.

The trick is to learn to call bullshit on yourself. Do you want to lose weight? Sure you do! Do you say to yourself, 'Oh, I will start once I empty out the cupboards and the fridge'? Bullshit. Or do you say, 'I will start when the weather gets warmer'? Bullshit. Or maybe you are waiting for your best friend to call you to join the gym together? Bulllshiiittt! Now is the time, not tomorrow, not later, not when your friend says he or she is ready, but now. Is your kitchen full of delicious treats that are no good for you? There is nothing stopping you from walking over to your cupboard and fridge right now and emptying anything that is not good for you into the bin. You might even have to go hungry for a night – if your goal is to lose weight then maybe this will help! Tomorrow morning you can go to the shops and buy the foods that you need for a healthy diet. More on diets later... But the point is that there is no physical barrier, no magic force holding you back from doing whatever it is that you want to do – other than the force in your mind. You can redesign anything in your life that you want to. Do you think it is not worth trying because you tried something else in the past and that didn't work? I was like this too. But this is just another bullshit excuse. We need to empower ourselves to understand that things are not always going to work. Just like a science experiment, some things will work, and some won't. We need to *experiment*. If a scientist gave up their research after trying something that didn't work, where would society be today?

I hope that by now the inspiration is starting to feel alive inside of you so that you can make the changes that you need to make. Yes throwing out all those chocolates, snacks and ice-cream will suck, I know (*it's the part of the path that you don't want to do but know you need to do it)*; but I can guarantee you that it's the first step to becoming the person you want to be. Do you ever look at people and feel envious? Well the only difference between you and them is that they woke up and said, 'You know what I am going to do this. I am going to make the first step, no matter how small, even if it's in the wrong direction. Either way it's ok because I am moving, and I will eventually move forward.' Well maybe they didn't actually say that... but they did actually live it! Whereas you may have sat there and complained about how unlucky you are or how lucky they are. It is time for all of us to learn that this is life. How many actors have failed to make it? I am sure that there are thousands of potential movie stars who are working office jobs, thousands of athletes who could have won a gold medal if the wind was blowing in a different direction the day that they went to junior trials, thousands of people who have missed out on their dreams just because of the way the cards fell. This is a part of life. Are you jealous of the movie star? Not really, you might just want their lifestyle. So why are you envious of someone who you personally know that has had a little success? We need to redesign the way our mind works to free us from envy and allow happiness for ourselves and others to flow.

Studies show that it takes 21 days to create a habit. If you make a change today, you literally could be a different person in 21 days' time. How good is that! Redesigning your mind could have an immense impact on your life and where you are going in less than a month's time. Have you ever had the feeling that a friend has changed? Maybe they found a new partner and a few weeks later you don't see them as much as you used to. Well that is because they made a new habit. Maybe it is not a good one, but after 21 days the habit has set in. Redesigning your mind will take effort. It will take time, but maybe not as much time as you first thought. As we move through this book I want you to think about some of the things you want to redesign in your life and why you want to do it. Challenge yourself to grow. Challenge yourself to throw out the things that no longer serve you. Challenge yourself to be responsible for your own life. I know that deep down you really do want to change and for this reason I know that you will get there if you give the process your all.

Looking back now, over the last six years of my life since that holiday to the US, it is remarkable to think about how much I have changed in my life. Looking back, I clearly think that starting a business was something I wanted to do to try and find more meaning in my life. Whilst I always wanted a business, I didn't really need to do it – it was more because I wanted to keep growing and growing, and my meaning was highly aligned to money and job success. Remember how I said I couldn't decide if I wanted to complete extra financial planning study or not? Well I finally decided NOT to cancel the course and I actually did finish it and managed to get a job as a financial planner. Recently I completed my Master of Financial Planning (while working full time). It's funny because I probably ended up doing the same amount of work and overtime that I would have done if I had my business; but because of a redesign of my thought processes, I am no longer thinking about work or creating anxious thoughts in my spare time. What I do outside of my working hours is now very different which helps make life much more manageable. As you read on you will find out more about what I have implemented to become the person I am today.

THE TEST

A few years ago I wanted to challenge myself and I booked a trip to Europe (for the first time) on my own (also for the first time). No one knew how much this meant to me to be able to face the challenge of going on another overseas holiday after the disastrous USA trip some years before. Things were going well, I had redesigned my life and I was really happy with where I was at; so why not plan a holiday on my own, to somewhere I had never been before, even further away than I had ever been – away from the sanctuary of my family and friends in the little old city of Adelaide. Just like anything exciting in life I got some people telling me that I was crazy, some saying that it will be fun, some scared for me and some wanting me not to do it. Maybe some of these people were jealous that I could decide to do this on my own but either way this was something that I had to do to prove to myself that I was able to do it. To prove that *I did like travel* and most importantly that *I was not scared!* It was time to put all I had learnt about anxiety and depression, and all my new tools, to the test and board a plane to Europe by myself.

So I was now on my way to Europe and at the back of my mind there was the fear that I would get sick again; the fear that I would lose my confidence again; the fear that I would have a shit time and regret it; the fear that I would fall back into anxiety or depression and undo all of my good work; and the fear that it wasn't worth it. *You can imagine what I was thinking when the Chicken dinner on the airplane came out!* My new bag of tools really helped me on this journey and as the trip went on I flourished and grew in confidence. I accepted my fears and dared myself to do more; to have more fun, to put myself out there, to explore, to get rejected, to f*ck up, to look like an idiot, to not care about what other people thought about me. I retained my confidence and yes, I went to Europe and I had the time of my life!

To experience travelling again and actually enjoy it was amazing. Some of you may not understand why this was a challenge, and others will totally understand the elation of what I felt when I overcame this challenge. The monkey was off of the back and it felt great. Yes, there were times of anxiety and when the trip ended I was somewhat depressed (who doesn't get depressed after the time of their life holiday), but this was easy to overcome with my new tools.

CHAPTER ONE – AN INTRODUCTION TO CHANGE

SHARING MY REDESIGNED MIND

On one of my final days on my holiday I took some time to reflect and enjoy the moment. I had a feeling of pure joy and happiness. A feeling where I knew I had tested myself and achieved so much. I was sitting on a beach in Greece and I had a moment to myself when I thought about the story that I mentioned earlier about searching for that beach in Paradise. There were times when I was at my lowest point, when I didn't know if I would ever find my beach. I reflected back to the moment when my dad showed how concerned he was for me, the pain I had felt, and the damage I had done to myself and those around me, when I just wanted to be happy again. I longed for a moment of freedom where I would be on a beach with nothing else on my mind other than enjoying the beach. Finally, I truly felt like I had found my paradise beach. I had to endure a journey of challenges to get there but it was well worth it. In a meditative sense I felt as if I was sitting there watching myself, happy with myself for what I had achieved. My spine was tingling with positive energy. I was in paradise and it was so worth it.

After some time reflecting and enjoying the moment, the thing I quickly learned about life is that even when we do find paradise, we then think about the search for the next paradise. Yes, this was great, and what a journey it had been, but now it was time to move forward again. I knew that there would be more challenges to come in life; some would be harder to get through than what I've been through already, but I knew that I had developed a resilience and set of tools that are going to keep me moving forward in a much better state than I would have in the past. Upon returning from my paradise beach I realised that I had to help others by sharing my story, empowering people to see that they can redesign their life too. I had to help those at the bottom of the barrel who were questioning whether or not there was a way out from anxiety and depression. I wanted people to come out of it just like I did. No one should ever feel alone or as if they can't make it; because if I can make it, you can too.

Upon returning from my European escapade I started my own mental health blog. *Remember how the man who moves mountains starts by moving a small stone?* I didn't know what to expect with the blog and I made sure that I put no expectation on myself or the pressure of 'success' – whatever that meant. After launching the blog on Facebook amongst my friends, I was amazed at how many people contacted me after the launch – noting their own challenges, their struggles, and their own stories. I was even more surprised at the fact that some of the people who got in touch with me about these challenges were people that I thought would never have problems with anxiety or depression. These were the strong ones, the ones who seemed to have their lives together. I had even been envious of some of them in the past. People were surprised at how passionate I was about mental health and that I actually dealt with the challenges of anxiety and depression to such an extent. This was the moment that I knew that I had to write a book about my story and share it with the world. Sharing my story with the world became my next fear that I had to face.

THE HIGHS AND LOWS

Everyone knows that life is full of highs and lows. And we all know that when we are low, things can feel really bad. Unfortunately, there is no way we can stop the lows in life. Someone will pass, something will go wrong in the economy or an earthquake might tear your house in half. Sometimes it is in your control and sometimes it is not. Either way – what we can learn to control is how we react to the situation and how low we go.

Let's say your lows currently look like the sad line on the graph below. When things get bad, they really suck. Maybe it happens too often as well. What we want to work on is creating a life that is more like the happy line where we are happy and content some of the time, down at other times but rarely do we fall into a deep depression. This graph below might represent one single day for you, but for me I find that it might represent a few months to a few years – where something happens in my life which could trigger a depressive state.

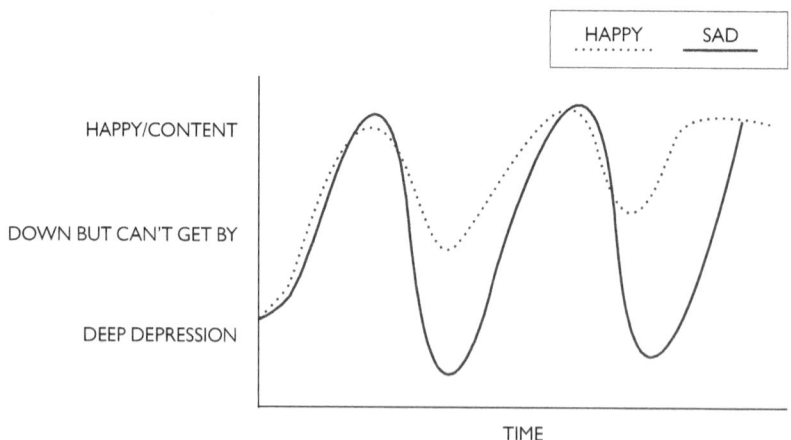

Now I could let depression set in and let myself sink lower by fuelling the negative thoughts, or I can acknowledge that I am heading downwards and make the necessary changes. Maybe I need to write out my thoughts and look for any cognitive distortions. Maybe I need to change my environment. Maybe I need to change my mindset. Maybe I need to 'act as if' things aren't as bad as they seem. There will be more on all of the tools that I use day in day out later, but for now I want you to understand that you are in control. You can always make a difference to how you feel; even if it is the slightest increment it will still make a massive difference.

We can't expect to be happy and content all the time. This is one of the causes of anxiety and depression. I used to want a perfect score, to avoid pain and unhappiness, but unfortunately life doesn't always go the way you want it to. I want you to draw what your graph looks like now and what you would like it to look like. Just having this as a visual will do so much for you. This graph will also help you tune into your feelings and emotions. You will be able to check in with yourself to see where you think you are on the graph at any point in time. Let's see if we can reduce the amount of lows and try to stop you from hitting rock bottom in the future. Things will suck at times but with the tools you implement from this book things won't suck as much or for as long.

As mentioned above, I still have times where I am pissed off or down, but what I focus on is what is in my control and how I can help bring myself back up (or put a floor on how low I will go). Good and bad times will come but it is about soaking up the positive vibes from the good times that will get us through the bad times. Have you ever had an awesome time that just flew by and then the next day you think back to how good it was? In the past I would let these moments slip by and then felt depressed in the days after because of how good those times were and I was no longer feeling that way. That's a double whammy! We must learn to be present, embrace the moment, and then let it go and be happy that it ever happened – not depressed that it is now gone.

THE TIME MACHINE

If I could go back and tell myself anything seven years ago on that plane, it would be, *'Don't worry Stef, just have a good time, it's all going to be okay. And even if it's not going to be ok, that's not for you to decide anyway. Let the universe take its course and you just enjoy the ride. And learn how to surf...'*

Since I don't have a time machine, I will look at the positives. If those challenges hadn't happened then I wouldn't have learnt what I have. I feel that I would have led a life focused on material things while worrying about what everyone else thought about me. Instead I have changed my tune and am now living a life according to what brings me happiness. Assuming that time machines will be available for sale on Amazon in 2025, and you could go back in time a few years just to give yourself some advice, what would you tell yourself? Would you change anything? Would you tell yourself to enjoy life? To follow your dreams.

Whatever you told yourself, it means you have learnt some things over time – which is a great thing! Since we can't time travel yet, I want you to think about what you would tell yourself now? Like if you were 30 years older than today, talking to yourself now, what would you say? This is your opportunity to go back in time, or more so go into the future and then have your future self give you some advice (kind of like Back to The Future). You now have the opportunity to tell yourself what your deepest dreams and desires are. You have the opportunity to give yourself the advice and wisdom you would most likely have passed on to someone else.

What did you say to yourself? Did things come up that you didn't expect? Were you kind to yourself? Either way it is now time to start your journey to redesign your life. It is time for you to listen to yourself. No longer will we run on autopilot and live to the beat of someone else's drum. Now is the time to make your own music by redesigning your mind and reaping the rewards of a positive mindset and a life that has your own special meaning.

THE PERSONAL TRAINER FOR THE MIND

One of the things I tried was to see a psychologist. Whilst it wasn't cheap and felt like I was sitting on the couch during an episode of Frasier (a classic 90's sitcom), the experience was invaluable. At first it was a challenge to open up because I felt like I knew what was wrong with me and that I could sort it out myself. Eventually I let the psychologist in and the task of redesigning my mind officially began. It took five or six sessions before something changed in me and I felt empowered to fight this journey on my own. At the time I thought that the psychologist had just guided me in the right direction but looking back now I know that I would never have had the will or skill to get started without his help. In one of my last sessions the psychologist suggested that I read some books about the mind and how other people have dealt with anxiety and depression – as he thought I was ready to start my own training. Not long after that I said goodbye (maybe just for now) as I was now a student of the mind and my test was to make myself feel better. I like to think that the psychologist knew exactly how I would react to his strategy and that I was the type of person that wanted to take this challenge on. Just the fact that I knew I could book in another session if I needed to gave me the comfort to move forward on my own. I was now empowered, full of confidence and ready to beat the challenges that lay in front of me. As a result of my time with the psychologist, my life and devotion to mental health would dramatically change. Many books would be read over the coming months and years which turned me into the person that I am today. The recommended reading list at the back of the book contains some of the books that helped change my life and how I think they may help you too. I have included a small review on each book to help you decide if the book is right for you.

Only now do I understand the importance of seeing a psychologist, especially in your darkest or most challenging times. The word 'psychologist' may have negative associations, but it is time this was redefined. Wouldn't it be great if we saw psychologists as personal trainers for the mind? They really are no different to a personal trainer in the gym as they work to personally change something in your life. A physical personal trainer trains you in the gym with weights and meal plans to help you lose weight and stay fit; whereas a psychological personal trainer will train your mind with the right tools and coping mechanisms to help overcome anxiety, depression, and build a positive mindset. How good does that sound? Maybe everyone would want to see a psychologist if we describe it that way. The psychologist (personal trainer for the mind) officially kick-started my positive mindset and helped me at a time when I needed it most. Find a personal trainer for your mind that you feel comfortable with and keep working with them for as long as you need to. Just remember that a psychologist is no different to a physical personal trainer in that you need to do your own work outside of the session to stay fit – the psychologist will just coach you along the way.

FEELING GOOD

Filled with the belief planted by my psychologist, I went home and Googled 'best books for anxiety and depression'. The first result was a book by David Burns – *Feeling Good: The New Mood Therapy (1980)*. I was happy that I was now using Google to search for books to fix my mindset instead of diseases that cause anxiety. David's book really opened my eyes to the belief that a positive mindset (or negative) can be created by how we wire our brain. His book is full of tools and techniques that will help you move from feeling down to feeling good.

How good would life be if you had only positive, happy thoughts coming into your head all day? Would there be any depression or anxiety if every thought you had was positive or happy? If you found out that you were going to die and the first thought that popped into your head was 'Oh well, at least I have lived a good life and I won't have to go to work on Monday' – then you wouldn't feel too bad! You might even smile at death (we have all been there on a Monday after holidays). However, our programmed thoughts on death make us feel sad and even anxious. This is all to do with the wiring of our brain and how you *frame* the information being presented. This is what Cognitive Behavioural Therapy (CBT) is all about. The way I see it is that our emotions are driven by the below process;

Event > Thoughts > Emotions

Something happens; you think whether it is good, bad or indifferent, and then you feel happy, sad, angry, depressed or anxious. That's it. We can't control a lot of what happens in life, but we can learn to program our thoughts which will lead to the right emotions. The positive or negative thoughts that you feed yourself will lead to the positive or negative emotions that you feel. It is important to remember that we don't want to stop any initial thoughts, but we can change how we react to the thought, and what rational responses we implement to our thoughts. We can also train our mind so that hopefully, after enough repetition, the initial thought is a positive one or a thought that leads to a challenge that you can overcome. I can tell you now that when you have a negative thought it is *NEVER* a good idea to tell that thought to go away or try and shut it out as it will only come back stronger and harder. Just like that bully we all knew back in high school. If we let the bully make fun of us and we have a laugh about it, the bully will eventually get bored and move on because he or she is not getting the reaction they are looking for. However, if we let it affect us and the bully sees it they will keep coming back for more. Our negative thoughts are the same. Accept the thought and let it pass without fighting it.

The Chinese talk about moving with the flow in life and bending like the willow tree. The Dao talk about going with the flow of life. If you are on a river, let the river take you down the tide; don't try and fight it as you might sink. Let the flow and current take you where you are going. Don't worry about whether the current will continue or not or get depressed about the fact that you are moving from one place to another or that you are not moving where you want to move, just acknowledge that you are moving, accept that you are moving, and let the flow of life take you along your own journey.

Hopefully by now you have started to open your eyes to different ways of looking at the world and you can see that the thoughts that you are empowering are going to determine your emotions.

WHAT DO YOU THINK?

It's time for a little activity. Grab a piece of paper and write down any negative thoughts that you had throughout the day. Underneath that negative thought I want you to rewrite how this thought could be seen as a positive. This is a way of starting to train your mind to think positively. A way to overcome a negative challenge. It will take time, so the sooner you start, the quicker your mind will start to develop the right thoughts. For example here is one of my latest ones;

That girl didn't show up for our date >> That's ok, if she couldn't show up to a first date then she wasn't going to be good enough for you anyway, and now at least you can go and meet up with your friends for a drink.

We want to train our mind to rationalise any negative thoughts with positive, rational thoughts. Once you are done, smile at the thought and have a laugh about it. I mean really, if a chick doesn't show up to a date, who wants to be with them anyway? Why would we let this bother us? Just like watching ourselves on a TV show we need to not take ourselves so seriously and have a laugh about it. By retraining our thoughts, we will get there eventually.

I was writing my thoughts out every day for at least 3 months but eventually it got easier and easier, and I had to write fewer thoughts as time went on. It's like you are learning a new language and I don't know anyone who can learn how to speak Italian in three weeks *(if you know someone who can teach me Italian in three weeks please send me their details)*.

AM I SAD, DEPRESSED, OR ANXIOUS?

It is important to recognise that there is a difference between feeling sad and something else such as feeling depressed. Sometimes our temporary sadness can develop into a long-term depression as a result of replaying the sad thoughts and causing additional pain. For example, if a loved one has just passed away you will be feeling sad. Relating this back to our emotions process let's take a look at this example in more detail.

1 Event >2 Thoughts >3 Emotions

1 Someone died >2 it's not fair. I miss them. I wish they were still here. What am I going to do without them in my life? What is the point of living? Why didn't I spend more time with them when they were alive? >3 Sadness, disappointment, depression

It is totally normal to grieve for someone and feel sadness, but after this initial grieving period we need to implement positive thoughts to help avoid any unnecessary depression. I know it's not easy to do but we have to reduce the negative loop of thoughts. Let's say that after an original set of thoughts like the above, after a period of grieving, you start implementing the thoughts as below;

1 Someone died >2 I was so grateful to have met this person. We shared some great experiences together. He really could make me laugh. Their life is over, and I will miss them, but I will always have them with me in my mind and in my heart. I will always be able to remember the good times. I am a better person because I met them >3 Grateful, content, maybe even happy?

You can see that our emotions are now much more positive after implementing positive thoughts of this negative event. This does not mean we have rose-coloured glasses and dismiss the loss of someone we love – but we grieve, accept the thoughts and then start to inject the positive thoughts instead of replaying the negative ones. Remember that we cannot stop the waves, but we can learn to surf.

UPDATE READY TO INSTALL

Just like when Apple makes you update to the latest IOS software (damn you Apple!) it is time to update our thought processes. Anyone reading this book has good hardware, that's like the computer or the CPU. You've read this book this far, so you have much better hardware than some of our ancestors did 10,000 years ago. Your mind has the right hardware that is capable of doing amazing things. The next part is the software – the IOS software and apps that you are loading on to your hard drive. I believe that much of the software that is loaded into our system is wrong. We think it is right, because that is all we know, but it is wrong. Throughout time there are numerous examples of massive amounts of people with the wrong 'software' installed. Think of the KKK's treatment of African Americans, Hitler and the Nazi party, and when all the guys thought it was cool to dye their hair platinum blonde (or was that just me?). All jokes aside, we can be programmed to believe that things are right, even when they are wrong. I believe this is what has happened to a lot of our thinking. We now look back at these events and think, 'How could this have happened', but the simple fact is that people were programmed to think a certain way. I am sure that some of the people who were involved in these travesties were good people who thought they were doing the right thing, but that's exactly the point. They had the wrong software which told them they were doing the right thing. The rest of the people involved were just dicks.

The good news is that you have the opportunity to update the software and that is what we are going to do. You can implement software that is inspiring, positive, and ready to deal with life's challenges. At the same time, we will delete our negative, outdated software that is clogging up our heads with shit.

Who gave you these inspirations to want money, a nice car, a nice house, a high status, to win, to get what you want, to be special, and everything else? Were we born with these dreams? I don't think so. Because if we were born 20,000 years ago, the dreams we have today wouldn't be possible. Our software has evolved over time and it is up to us to decide if we want to go with what society has loaded into our minds or upload our own software. It doesn't mean we have to throw these dreams away, but it means that we rewrite what our real dreams are and focus on the present – not just on whether we get there or not.

One of the key steps to changing your software is to acknowledge that you want to change. By the end of this book (if not already) you will be ready to implement the actions and behaviours that will help you redesign your mind and your life. You will be on your way to practicing a mindset and trail of thoughts that are positive, uplifting and constructive. You will have a mindset that helps you smash anxiety, beat depression and embrace the positive.

CHAPTER TWO
HOW SOCIETY HAS SHAPED OUR LIVES

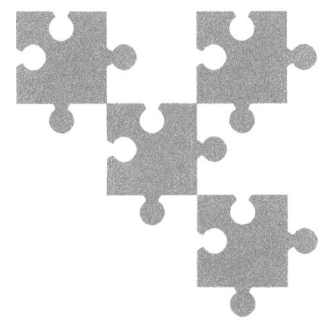

Let's go back 20,000 years to the pre-agricultural revolution days where life was all about the collective. People lived in simple sheltered structures within small clans of 25 to 50 people (Dorey, 2018). The members of the clan would work together and share their efforts for the benefit of the clan. On most days the men would hunt mammoths while the women would prepare meals, forage and look after the children. The clan was a collective society without individual possession. Everyone in the clan would have lived to the same standard (maybe with the exception of the clan leader). A clan member would have enjoyed shelter, food, water and entertainment with the rest of the group. There were no 70-inch TV's, broadband internet, sports cars, travel plans, new iPhone plans, restaurants, expensive toys, big houses, big mortgages, savings accounts or social media to compare your happiness with everyone else's.

Your life was the community and there were no choices as to what you did with your 'money' or discretionary time. Things were relatively simple. I'm sure that sometimes a few of the men in the camp got pissed off with each other – but no doubt after a punch up or fight to the death, life probably went back to normal. In my research of these times, I have found no evidence of mental illnesses such as anxiety and depression. You may argue that life back then was unfulfilling. Maybe it was. Maybe it was just different. And what is unfulfilling about hanging out with friends and family all day, playing games, not having deadlines to make, or traffic jams to sit in? What is unfulfilling about enjoying most of your days relatively carefree? Maybe it seems like an unfortunate life, but maybe it seems this way to us because we know a different life. But maybe it is our life that is unfulfilling? Maybe a life where having to work for five days out of seven days, every week for most of your life, only to spend most of your money on paying bills and mortgage repayments is unfulfilling?

ISLAND OF PARADISE

An interesting read on alternative ways of life is *Mastering Your Hidden Self: A Guide to the Huna Way* (A Quest Book) (1985) by Serge Kahili King. The book talks about some of the Huna teachings and ways of life. What I found most interesting was that there is a small community on an untouched island that is free of technology and interaction with the outside world. There is no record of these people ever experiencing depression or anxiety. How is it that this tribe in the middle of some untouched island has never suffered from depression? They have literally no possessions other than some basic tools and shelter, no money, no travel plans, no big weddings – yet they are totally happy and content? We have gadgets, cars, endless entertainment, more friends and people we know – yet we become depressed and anxious and need to read self-help books. Society has programmed us with the wrong 'software'.

Whilst today there is still some sense of community, it is nothing like the past. Money, possession and technology have decreased the need and want for a community existence. We have now become the individual. Even if we live in a very close family we still all have our own goals, identities, bank accounts, and live our own lives. The need to constantly achieve and be the best was something that I fell for. I consistently had to have my name up in lights, or be making more money, or adding another achievement to the list. In a community 20,000 years ago, I might have aspired to be tribe leader. Life was about being present, being in the moment, just as the other animals on this earth do. Life wasn't about trying to tick off as many goals as possible, or the pressures of having to live up to a certain expectation, or the desire for more. Life was about living and that was it.

HOW SOCIETY HAS CONDITIONED OUR MIND

So let's think about this; about 60 to 100 years ago there were wars, great depressions and poverty. There were migrants moving all over the world in the search for a better life. This resulted in a lot of people having to start again. I have been told that one of my great grandparents back in Italy had a lot of wealth and was well established in their community – however when my Nonno (grandpa) returned after being lost amongst wars and other things, his grandfather had started a new family and disowned him. I can only imagine how my Nonno must have felt, but he pushed on and moved on to the search for a better life. He eventually found his way down to Adelaide, Australia, and when he found her, asked my Nonna (grandmother) to marry him. They had nothing, building a life from hard work and a lot of sacrifice. Most migrants came to these countries with no possessions other than the clothes they were wearing. Our parents were brought up in hard working, capitalist countries, where their efforts would hopefully result in 'a better life'. They wouldn't even dream of having riches or a special life like some of us do today. Their children were the baby-boomer generation. Many of these children were brought up with a strong set of values and told to work hard, do their best, save money, buy a house, start a family, and enjoy a better life than their parents did.

Next came my generation, the Millennials. By now our parents had accumulated some wealth due to the hard work set up by their parents. This generation is the first to see a large portion of the population fitting into the upper-middle class. These are the people that aren't 'rich' but have enough to live a good life. Most of the Millennials have been brought up watching TV and are now on social media. Their minds are conditioned by what they see on TV and the internet. They believe money is cool, and fame is even cooler. Millennials are conditioned to think that they need these things to be happy. Life is now about being cool, popular, special, unique, smart and beautiful– way more than it ever was in the past. Because of our upper-middle class parents, more Millennials are able to go to university. With more opportunity comes way more pressure to achieve. Life has changed so dramatically in the past 40 or so years that we really have no idea how much we have been influenced by society's pressures. Unlike the tribe environment 20,000 years ago, we now all aspire to live the life of the rich and famous.

As technologies evolved and changed, we all had to change and evolve. Cars, televisions, phones, mobile phones, computers, iPhones, internet, big screen TV's and holidays all became part of our desires. Even if you go back only 100 years ago there were none of these choices. If you were a millionaire back in the early 1900's there was only so much you could buy. There were no planes to fly, sports cars to drive, and social media to show it all off. Flash forward to today and our choices on how to spend our time and money are endless. Our choices have increased but our resources (money and time) have decreased. Our range of choice has created a lot of the pressure that exists today. Remember that the little community in the middle of nowhere has no depression or anxiety; yet here we are with all the luxuries and safeties of the modern world and we feel like shit. We have so much choice that it becomes difficult to even make the choice in the first place.

WHAT 'THINGS' ARE IMPORTANT?

Big business and the evolution of society has dramatically changed how we behave and what 'things' are important to us. I'm not a flower throwing hippie – but I do believe that big businesses have significantly influenced how we behave on a day to day basis. There are thousands of examples but here are just a few to get you thinking.

I know that marriage has a different meaning for different people; but it would be safe to say that marriage is largely based on love and commitment. For a long period of time, marriage went without the need for expensive wedding rings and lavish wedding ceremonies. A wedding has always been about two people, who are in love, celebrating their commitment to each other. This has changed in the last century. Society has influenced our belief that no expense should be spared on a wedding. It is not uncommon to hear that a certain amount of money *should* be spent on a wedding ring. Depending on whom you speak to; 1 month's, 2 months' or even 6 months' salary should be spent on the ring alone! Why does the price tag on a wedding ring dictate how much we love each other? Has society influenced us to think that this is something that is now important?

As discussed earlier the Australian dream involves owning your own home and having a nice car to match; two cars preferably. Have we been influenced by big business and their new car commercials? Have we been conditioned to think that 'the new car smell' will bring us happiness? Do we see other people with their new car or new home and think 'I want that' without seeing the full picture, which might include large mortgage repayments and financial stress?

Why do we need the latest iPhone? I mean, seriously, Apple; paying $1,500 for a new phone that has a slightly higher resolution than my existing iPhone (which still works perfectly) is kind of silly. Has Apple influenced us to think that having the latest iPhone will make us happy? Of course they have! Big businesses spend billions of dollars on researching how they can tap into our minds and make us think that buying their product will make us happy.

What 'things' are really important to you? Why is it that previous generations could get by with just the food on the table and the love of their family, and our generation needs to have all of these 'things' to be happy? When you are on your death bed, will you be thinking about how good your life was because of an expensive wedding ring, nice house, flashy car, or timely iPhone upgrade? Or will you be flashing back to all the priceless memories of love and happiness that were brought to you by your family, friends and life experiences?

Having a desire for all of these 'things' is a great cause for our negative thinking. Relating this to my life – the bar was continuously raised and no matter what I achieved the next goal was ready to replace my latest achievement. I finished university; great, now get a good job. I got a good job; great, now buy a nice car. Bought a nice car; great, now buy a house. I bought a house; great now buy another one. Most of these pressures came from my own thoughts, but other people would always add to the pressure without even trying. Regardless of your achievement, people are always asking you 'what next'? This relentless pressure to continuously achieve can become a burden.

How many of us have received a promotion and pretty soon after we are stretching ourselves financially by taking on another debt? Even though you have only just started the new role, and don't even know if you are going to like it, you take on a debt based on your new income. From here the pressure builds. If you start to realise that this job is not for you, or you want to step down, it may already be too late. *How will I make the mortgage repayments if I quit my job or ask to step down? Oh no, I would have to sell the house!*

Technology was developed with the view of making our lives easier, more fulfilling and to save us time. But does it really do any of these things? How long do we spend on our smart phones? What about all the hours we spend on our computer at work? This is another thing that makes me laugh. We say that technology was meant to make work *easier*, but all that happens is companies use the technology to reduce staff and increase profits and keep the workload the same on the remaining employees. It's perfect business, but it's not great for us as individuals.

What about work anyway? Who decided that eight hours a day is the normal amount of work required? And who said that if you can't finish your work in eight hours that you should work unpaid overtime? Why has society made these rules that seem to challenge what we truly want to do with our lives? Sometimes we forget that we work to live and not live to work. So why do we spend so much of our time at work, only to come home and often think about it there too! If you work eight hours a day, as a guess the average amount of time getting ready for work and travelling to work might be 45 minutes each way. So that's 90 minutes a day, plus one-hour lunch break when you are still somewhat tied to your work as you can't venture too far. So we dedicate an estimated 10.5 hours of our life just arranging our income for the day. Why is this fair? If eight hours per day is 40 hours per week, well then why didn't whoever was in charge at the time decide that we could work ten hours per day for four days per week and enjoy a three-day weekend? Why would this not be normal if someone requested it now? Why do we stay back at work without receiving overtime? Would your boss be as lenient on you if you came in 30 minutes late every day?

This is just an example of how society has shaped what we think is normal and acceptable. If you were born 100 years ago, or in 100 years' time, the way you live your life would be different. You cannot change society overnight, but you can start by redesigning yourself.

Remember how I talked about your thought processes and your 'software'? Your software is loaded and bombarded daily with success and happiness being awarded to the winners, rich, poplar, famous and good looking. It plants a seed in us 'normal' people to want some of these things. I have seen it in everyone and most of all I have seen it in myself. I wanted to win. I wanted to be the best, the richest, the smartest, the one everyone looked up to, maybe even famous – the whole lot. Society planted ideas in my head of what I needed to live a happy life and I believed it. The ideas grew into a monster. They became a major cause for my anxiety and depression and it had to stop. One of the thoughts I had to program into my head was to accept that it is ok to be average. It is ok to not be a winner, rich, popular, famous, good looking, forever young, special or wanted.

To be honest when I first started toying with the idea of being average it hurt. My whole life I had been told that I was special, that I was going to be something. I had achieved again and again and I felt that I was entitled to being successful and rich. I had to pull a lot of these roots out that grew from small seeds and plant my own seeds of positive, free-flowing attitudes to help cultivate the life I wanted to live. Just like ripping out the weeds in an uncared-for garden, it takes time. Some of these weeds will grow back. We need to keep pulling them and planting the right seeds to continue to cultivate our garden. My redesigned mind greatly changed how I felt about myself. I no longer had the pressure of needing to be someone or something special. We are all someone. It doesn't matter if you are rich, famous, or seen as special. Our minds may take time to adjust to this fact because society constantly conditions us to think that these things bring us happiness. Everyone we see on the stage, in the spotlight, or on TV has these things and we are trained to believe that they are happy. But unfortunately *(fortunately?)* these things do not bring long lasting happiness. The sooner we accept this, the sooner we can commence our journey to proven, lasting happiness without the need for this superficial oasis.

ARE YOU HAPPY?

Are you happy right now? What does it even mean to be happy? Write down a few lines on what happiness means to you. Happiness starts from your thoughts and not from what happens to you. 'Bad' events are going to happen in life; however it is the thoughts that we choose to encourage and cultivate that will lead to our emotions. Happiness does not come from what Jack Smith thinks about you, but from what you think about yourself. For example if Jack Smith comes past your house and says, 'You look like you've put on weight', would you get pissed off? Probably. Has Jack pissed you off? No. You've pissed yourself off. *What?!* Yes, that is right. Jack just said something, regardless of his intentions and you have decided to let this piss you off. You have accepted that what someone else says about you is how you determine your happiness. Is this how you want to live your life? According to what someone else says or thinks about you?

Regardless of whether you are overweight or not, you could laugh at this comment (and Jack will probably laugh with you) and you could make a joke about him (or yourself being overweight) too. But if you take offense to this, then are you being harsh on yourself? You are pissing yourself off for no reason. What we must do is rewrite our thoughts and implement the seeds of the thoughts that we want to come up next time this happens. You can choose to ruminate on the negative thoughts, or you could plant positive thoughts and maybe a goal to lose weight! What has someone said to you in your life that has pissed you off? How could you rewrite these negative thoughts you had? And what new, positive, light-hearted, happy, or positive thoughts can you implement instead? Trust me when I say it will take time for these thoughts to take hold, but it will happen.

POST. LIKE. SHARE. REPEAT.

Social media has changed our lives and how we interact with friends and those around us. Only 20 years ago much of what we do now on a day to day basis didn't even exist! We now use the internet on our mobile phones to 'like' photos of people on our Instagram accounts – often without even knowing who they are. Social media has influenced how happy we think we are compared to everyone else. 30 years ago you may have envied your friends when they showed you their photo album of holiday snaps but the album would then have been put away and your envy would be over. Flash forward to today. You most probably start the day by picking up your phone and scrolling through your Facebook feed. Depending on your age you're likely to be bombarded with your friends' recent achievements, and your friends of friends' achievements. Let's say you have 500 friends on Facebook and assume that on average each of them post something happy or special about ten times per year (so that's 5,000 posts that you view each year of someone else's highlights, or 13.7 posts per day). Now this sounds a bit technical but I am sure you agree that 13.7 posts a day of other people's successes and highlights is making us feel like we are missing out.

Upon waking up on this particular day you have seen that Sarah's two year old learnt to walk, Jenny has just made a new friend called Sergio the bartender in Barcelona, Jim got engaged to Ben, Jack got a promotion, Steve is going away for the weekend, Leah enjoyed an awesome dinner at a top restaurant last night, and Ellie is posting memories of her trip to Thailand two years ago (even though this is old news your mind still recognises this as something good that happened to someone else). Facebook fills your feed with advertisements based on what they think you really need, which reminds you that flights to Japan are only $800 return. Without even getting out of bed your mind is already full of great things you are missing out on. You want those flights to Japan to make your life better. You want a lot of the things that everyone else has shown in their highlight reel. You conclude you have nothing, or that you are unlucky, or that you are not worthy of a relationship, or that you need those flights to Japan to be happy. What type of emotions are these thoughts of loss and missing out going to lead to?

Even if your life is good, and even if your highlight makes you feel good, you still have seen 13.7 other posts of good things and your mind starts to want more. We don't acknowledge that this is just a highlight reel and that there are often sacrifices or consequences for these highlights. We see that Grace went on a holiday to Europe; but we don't see that she has a massive credit card debt that she had to get Mum and Dad to help pay for when she got home. We see that Adam and Linda bought a new dream house and look like they are living the dream; but we don't see their bank statement showing that they have a huge mortgage and Linda is lying in bed awake at night wondering how they are going to make the mortgage repayments. Social media does not show the 'behind the scenes' or the disclaimers of every happy post – you only see the glory moments. Our mind may think that we have to struggle through our challenges, maybe a job we aren't happy with, or bills to pay, or a challenging family member – while everyone else is living the good life. The funniest part about all of this is that some of your friends scroll through their feed and think the same thing about you! If you watched your own 'highlight reel' over the past few years, no matter how challenging your life may have been, I am sure that your social media account will show that you had a great time. I know this because I did it myself. When I was in my darkest days I wasn't posting photos of myself lying on the couch struggling with life. If I managed to make it out to an event I would be tagged in some photo with my friends and everyone would think it was all good. There was nothing to say that I ever went through depression or anxiety, and this is another reason why we can never tell who is actually going through these challenges with their mental health. This is another reason why we need to be more open, accepting, and inviting to those experiencing anxiety and depression.

We need to learn to stop measuring our normal lives against someone else's highlight reel. We need to acknowledge that we don't know what ups and downs that person is going through. Maybe we can spend less time on social media checking up on what everyone is doing? Maybe as a collective we can stop posting less highlights and start posting more average points of our lives? I know it sounds silly, doesn't it! But why not? Why not show the world that we are average, normal people and we don't care if we haven't perfectly filtered our photo to maximise the amount of likes? Why don't we start spending more time being *present* and not on our phones?

It is time for us to *stop* idolising these images of a perfect world because these things do not bring happiness even if you had them. Everything on social media is all about the image or the visual. If everything we perceive about life is through the lens of our eyes and compared to the perfect visual of others, then of course you are going to feel depressed, anxious or disappointed. We need to remember that even though these people look like they have the perfect life – they don't. Some of them are even less happy with the riches and fame and would much rather be like you. We need to redesign how we use social media by using it as a tool, as something to help enhance our lives and not something that makes us feel small.

HOW MANY LIKES DID YOU GET?

Have you ever posted something on social media that received a huge amount of likes or positive comments? How good did it feel? Did you feel great as the number of likes and activity soared past your usual number of likes? It feels great for me! We love this feeling and receiving a 'like' is just a way to boost our ego. Simon Syneck is a great speaker on the effects of our own behaviours, and in particular the effects of social media. In one of his videos he talks about studies on what happens to the brain when we receive a 'like' on Facebook. As a result of the 'like' we receive a hit of dopamine which also results in endorphins being released throughout the body. We 'like' this. The catch is that every time we get a hit, we want more, and we want to feel that same feeling again and again. We don't even realise that this is happening as we are on auto-pilot thanks to our 'software'.

Some of you may be thinking that you aren't as affected by social media as everyone else, and you don't even post regularly. Yes, you may not be as bad as the rest of us, but you still live in this society and you are part of the collective. You still form part of the socially connected community. And unless you have no TV, no smart phone, no internet, no computer and no radio – then you are connected to the external world of social media in some form. The way things are going I expect that social media is going to become ever more intertwined in our lives in the future. I still like social media; however I have totally redesigned the way I use it. No longer do I need it to gratify me or do I allow it to get me down – now I see it as a way of keeping in touch with friends and family around the world and having fun. I know this was the aim of social media in the first place, but the point is you need to ask yourself if you have been affected in some way. Social media played a part in my anxiety of wanting to stay ahead and keep up with everyone else – which eventually led to depression when I found out that I wasn't as special as I thought. Social media is going to continue to evolve and try to play a part in shaping what we think, what we buy, when we buy it, what is hot, what is not, and everything else in between. It will be up to us to decide if we want to be told what our lives need to look like to be happy or if we can decide this for ourselves.

ENTITLEMENT

Society has led us to believe that we are all entitled to certain things such as civil rights, healthcare, freedom of speech, rising wages and to be treated fairly. These all seem like basic human rights; but do these really exist or is it just a fragment of our imagination? Think about it. Maybe you believe that we should be entitled to some of these things but not all of them. Either way let's ask ourselves if these same entitlements apply to a Sudanese girl living in a war-torn peasant village who has no money, no police, no structure? What are her civil rights? Why are we so special that because we are born in a Western Society in the 21st century we are entitled to these things? The answer is because we grew up with this *expectation*. We grew up being told that everyone is equal and that everyone is entitled to the same basic needs – which is a load of shit.

Everyone has won the life lottery with existence as the prize. But how much you won depends on many factors. Let's say that you are a Millennial and given that you are reading this book it means that you are most likely more educated than billions of people that were born and died before you. How would you feel if you were transported back to the 1800's, with no electricity and no iPhone? What about if you were still a Millennial but were born in a third world country, with no parents, no food and nothing to your name. Is it right that because we were born in a different place and time to someone else we are more entitled? We are already so lucky just to be living at such an advanced time in such an advanced place. Telling someone from the 1800's that you could buy a TV to watch endless amounts of entertainment wouldn't have been believable, and yet here we are in the 21st century where we think that televisions and Netflix are just one part of our entitlements.

To be honest with you we are not entitled to anything. The universe flows whichever way it likes regardless of what we want, demand or expect. If you graduate with a Uni degree, you are not entitled to a good job. You have a better chance of a good job – but it is not guaranteed. If you work hard all your life, you are not entitled to more wealth than the next person. The chances are that if you work hard and save all your life, you will have more wealth than the next person – but it is not guaranteed. The world has never been this old before and we, as a society, have never been as advanced as we are now. With each new day the world ventures further and further into unchartered territory which means that whatever worked yesterday may not work today (and vice versa).

We cannot let our thoughts of what happened in the past set our expectation on the future. Maybe the person who went to Uni will end up in a field that has been replaced by robots? Maybe the person who had worked hard and saved their whole life will lose it all in one bad investment. We can make our lives a lot easier if we remove our entitlements and expectations. I know it's not easy because I was one of the most entitled people who set the highest expectations. If I worked hard – I was entitled to success. If I made an important decision, it was expected to be the right one. All that entitlements and expectations create are unnecessary pressures which cause anger, frustration, envy and disappointment when things don't go to plan. These pressures ultimately led to anxiety and depression. I had to evolve.

Removing these expectations can have some other positive effects too. When you are in a deep depression, even getting out of bed can feel like climbing a mountain. Your mind may think that it is going to be like this forever and there is no point going on. However, by removing the expectation that things are going to be this way forever, you free your mind to allow yourself to get better in your own time. Your future is not written and set by a false expectation that your mind created.

It does not mean by removing these expectations and entitlements that we no longer look to achieve our goals in life. Instead we can pursue these goals without the burden of expectation. We can be proud of our achievements, but we do not become entitled to more recognition, more wealth, or more happiness than the next person. I have never been as motivated and driven as I am today – but I have removed the expectation that this drive is going to result in success. I have removed the entitlement that because I work hard and have more qualifications than I used to have, that it means I will be more successful. By pursuing my goals and ambitions without expectation and entitlement, I can live free, without the burden of whether my pursuits will result in success or failure. You can do this too.

One day, if you're lucky enough, at a very old age you will get to say goodbye to the people you love. At this moment I am sure that you will look back at your life and wish that you could live it all over again. We can empower ourselves to be present and start enjoying life right now by letting go of the expectation that our life will be like this forever. Life is full of great and not so great moments. Depression is just one of those moments in time that you need to endure to get to the good times. Many of life's challenges are out of our control. We need to acknowledge and accept that we cannot control much of what happens to us, with the view that we can learn to cultivate a mindset that will help us get through these challenges. We can't stop the waves, but we can learn to surf.

KNOWLEDGE OR WISDOM

In recent years I have read books on happiness, depression, anxiety, and studied ways of life including Buddhism, Confucianism and Daoism. I have researched a great deal of knowledge on how to live a happy life; but I am still working on the *wisdom* of how to live a happy life. Do you know the difference between knowledge and wisdom? When I was younger I thought I had all the knowledge in the world. I remember saying to my dad one day when I was about 13, 'Dad, I think I know all there is to know about life'. I remember he laughed at me and said, 'Yeah, sure you do'. I love the audacity of my thoughts at the time, but it is now obvious that ignorance is bliss and unfortunately this ignorance played a part in forming anxiety and depression. The thing is that even if I did have some knowledge (which I didn't), I had no wisdom. I hadn't *lived* through all of the things that I thought I knew. This is the difference between knowledge and wisdom; knowledge is knowing and wisdom is living. It pertains to someone who has been there and tasted the experience. No matter how knowledgeable you are, you cannot be wise until you have experience. If I said here is the recipe and ingredients to make a 12-tier cake with 15 blends of chocolate and cream you would have all the *knowledge* you need to make the world's best cake – but what do you think it would look like on your first attempt? Yes some of you master-chefs may think that you can do it on your first go, but most likely you are going to cock it up. You had all the knowledge, but none of the wisdom.

Wisdom *takes time*. Wisdom cannot be bought, stolen or given away. Yes, it can be shared in the form of knowledge, but again your own wisdom will only come through your own experiences. And this is exactly why I was a classic 'know it all' who had lived through none of this and had no idea of how hard life was going to hit when it wanted to. This is why all of the knowledge and information you read in my book and every other book you read will only help you if you put something into practice. This is why people who have never experienced anxiety or depression have no idea what it is like to be anxious or depressed – until they experience it for themselves and wish they never had.

I know I am still relatively young, but relating this back to what was said before, what is 'young'? I am 30 and in my field of work I am considered 'young'.

But if I go and see my ten-your-old little cousins, they think that I am 'old' (*thanks guys*). This is all based on relative perception. None of it is true because I cannot be young and old at the exact same time! Do you have to be old to be wise? Of course not! You could be 21 and have gone through so much in your life that you are wiser than a 40-year-old. I know some 'old' people in their 50's that couldn't provide advice to a 10-year-old, let alone be considered wise! So, let's become wise in our thoughts and understand that good times will come and go, meaning that we can always remain centred no matter where we are at.

REMOVING EXPECTATIONS

Do you think that if we removed all of our expectations, we would also remove much of our mental pain? Most of our sadness, anger, disappointment, anxiety, and depression comes from the expectations we place on something in our lives. If we remove these expectations then maybe we can remove a lot of our mental pain. If I am nice to a friend, I expect them to be nice to me. If I stay back at work, my boss should be happy. If a date went well, the girl will like me. However in the real world if you stayed back at work, you might still miss out on that promotion; or if a date went well, you might find out that the girl has decided to get back with her ex; or that friend you were nice to doesn't really care about you. The real world doesn't follow our expectations and as a result we need to learn to remove expectations – unless you are happy to be disappointed.

Are you pressured by others to find a partner? If you remove the expectation that you need to get married or find a partner to find happiness, you will come to the realisation that your happiness is not reliant on finding a partner. If it happens it happens; if not, well you didn't expect anything anyway, meaning you are no longer vulnerable to depression from this expectation. We all know of many couples that aren't happy together, so why do we fixate on the need to be with someone to be happy? As a young Australian with an Italian background, I know that much of this expectation comes from our traditions, family and friends. If there is such an expectation to find a partner because everyone else has, does this mean that there is also an expectation that we will need to start thinking about divorce when some of the other couples are getting divorced? Of course not! We need to learn to remove the pressure of having to live up to the expectations of others. This goes for any of your goals in life where we strive towards it – but cannot burden ourselves with the expectation of when, or even if it will happen.

You have the power to redesign your mind and work on cultivating a mindset that you want and that will deal with your life's challenges. It doesn't mean that you will never feel anxious or depressed but it will mean that the changes you put in place today will better prepare you to get through it. We have all been influenced by society in one way or another and it is now up to us to acknowledge that maybe we have been a little too influenced; maybe we do care a little bit too much about what others think; and most importantly, believe that we have the power to change it all.

CHAPTER THREE
REDEFINING DEPRESSION

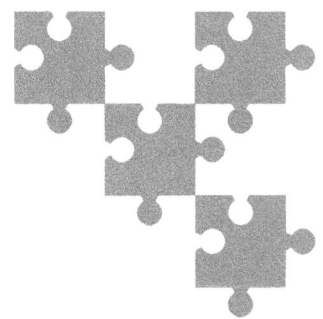

WHAT IS DE-PRESSION

Over the years there have been different ways to define and treat depression. Situational depression, clinical depression, deep depression, major depression, and melancholia are just a few to note. Whatever the technical term for depression, we still cannot clearly define what causes it and how to overcome it. It is believed that it is a complex mix of your mindset, environment, personal experiences and genetics. The role each of these items plays in depression is still not certain. One thing I am sure about is that depression does not define who you are. You may be going through depression, but it is not a label you carry for the rest of your life.

Just as we talked about how the island that has been untouched by Western Civilisation has no record of anxiety or depression in their community, we know that our environment must play a part in why we feel anxious or depressed. Because of this it is important to remember that no two people are the same – we all share different stories, genetics and experiences which means that what might work for me might not work for you. I am talking about depression from my point of view which may be very different from your world. Whatever you try, just remember to keep trying different things because maybe it will be the cumulative build-up of all the things that you have tried over time that helps get you through depression. Hang in there, things will get better.

De-pression as I like to spell and define it; is basically a feeling of deflation or not being pumped up. You are like a football that is low on air. Everyone gets a little deflated at times and we just have to find a way to pump ourselves back up. Sometimes we are more than just deflated, we are fully flat – which I believe is when you are depressed. Anyone who has ever been depressed knows how challenging it can be. Being depressed can be like trying to run a marathon with unbearable weights strapped to your legs and shoulders. Any form of depression will have an adverse effect on your friendships, family relationships, work, health, performance and enjoyment of life.

When I first went through depression I felt as if I was alone. I felt weak for letting it happen to me. Now that I have my mental health blog it is amazing how many people open up to me about how they too have been depressed. Often, they feel depressed because something in their life is not the way it *should* be. There might be a sense of loss, a sense of regret, or a belief that the future is already written with nothing but pain ahead. They might wish they did this, or wish they did that. Sometimes people don't even know why they are depressed. This can be challenging because you don't know what to work on or why you are feeling this way. I can relate to this with my first bout of depression when I wasn't even aware (or accepting) of what depression really was. After seeing common trends in so many people (including myself), I now believe that our negative thoughts make depression worse than it needs to be.

Often when we are producing negative thoughts we have low energy and feel tired, sick or not 100%. You are not physically ill because of an illness; you are physically ill and low on energy because of your depression. No, you are not depressed because you aren't sleeping well – you are not sleeping well because you are depressed. You aren't depressed because you are craving junk food; you are craving junk food because you are depressed. This is why a lot of people (including myself) reach for the bucket of ice cream (yes bucket*)* when times are tough. We are burning so much energy struggling, thinking, and stressing that our body just wants the naughty stuff.

Depression is not something that you can 'have', 'own', or can physically see attached to a person. Whilst there are things you can do to reduce the chances of or severity of depression, we do know that there is no 100% preventative measure to protect yourself against depression. Depression can be felt by all ages and by people from different ways of life. What may be considered a 'good' event by you may be seen as a depressive event for someone else. For example having a child may be seen as a joyous event for one person, an anxiety forming event for another and a depressive forming event for another. For this reason, regardless of whether genetics or brain chemistry play a part in depression, I believe that any negative thought patterns will enhance feelings of depression.

Sometimes in what is known as situational depression, there is a trigger or event that leads to negative thoughts, resulting in negative emotions. A common example is breaking up with a partner;

Break up with partner (event) > Life sucks, I will never find anyone, I wasted years of my life, I am not worthy of someone etc (thoughts) > Sadness, loss, fear, worry, depression, anxiety (emotions)

CHAPTER THREE - REDEFINING DEPRESSION

Breaking up with a partner is just an event in your life and not what caused you to feel depressed. Your thoughts are what caused you to feel depressed. Imagine that, after breaking up, you had planted and cultivated seeds of positive thoughts and allowed the negative thoughts to go by, you may not have felt as depressed. For example;

Break up with partner (event)> Life has it's challenges but I will manage, I might find someone one day but for now I can enjoy being single, I enjoyed my time with my partner and now it is time to move on, I know that I am worthy and have a lot of love to give, and for now I will love myself and have fun. At least I can go out with my friends more often, and won't have to sit through another episode of Married at First Sight (thoughts) > Opportunity, reflective positivity, ready for the new chapter, sad that is over but happy that it happened - limited anxiety and limited depression before moving on (emotions)

We love seeing something like this in a movie, don't we? Girl breaks up with guy, guy is depressed, guy eventually moves on and succeeds at his passions, guy falls in love with another girl who is attracted to him because of his passions, now the ex-girlfriend wants him back but he sees her for being the shallow person that he didn't want to be with anyway. You can be that person, the one who gets on with life! With any 'bad' event in life, you can decide to move on and cultivate positive thoughts to create an energy that will lead to new opportunities. Working on your thought processes will change how you perceive events in your life and help reduce or remove situational depression.

Yes, you may feel physically ill; yes, you may be low in energy and yes, you may have negative thoughts flying into your head. However, all of these things do not mean that you are sentenced to a lifetime of depression. With the right thoughts and behaviour much of these depressive side effects will ease off or even disappear. With my own story, I had all the psychosomatic (don't worry I had to Google this word too) symptoms of anxiety and depression, including stomach aches, headaches, neck pain and dizziness. I was in such denial that these physical symptoms could be brought on by anxiety and depression that I spent a great deal of time on Google and attending doctors' appointments trying to figure out what was wrong with me. Now I understand that these symptoms were retriggered by my body's alarm system which was trying to tell me that I needed to change, and I was too ignorant to believe it. Eventually I learnt that these symptoms will not go away until you solve the root cause of your anxiety and depression. Working on your thoughts is going to help you release yourself from these depressive and anxious feelings and achieve more lasting happiness. I know that it is more challenging for some but that is just like anything in life. Some people are naturally smarter while others have to spend more time studying. Some people have beautiful bodies without trying, others have to spend time in the gym. Your mindset is no different to these challenges. There is nothing stopping you from hitting the 'mental gym' and creating and cultivating a positive mindset for yourself. With what is known as situational depression, you can choose to stay deflated and de-pressed or you can pump yourself back up and feel better than ever.

Sometimes the depression becomes part of your life for no definitive reason. You wake up one day and wonder what happened to you. Yesterday everything was great and today you are a shell of who you used to be. Like I mentioned before, this could be even more challenging than situational depression because you are not sure what to work on first. Often there may be an underlying reason that may be hidden away in the depths of your mind which is causing your depression – however you might not even be aware of it. This is why as I mentioned before, seeing a psychologist (personal trainer for the mind) can be invaluable in helping you uncover any underlying reasons for your anxiety or depression. Remember not to let depression define who you are and that you can always work to improve your situation, regardless of where you are today.

MEDICATION AND YOUR HEALTH

It is important that you work with your doctor and those around you in a way that is best for you. Remember that this is your life and it is up to you to decide how you want to live it. I know many people who rely on medication to help them live a happy, healthy lifestyle and there is nothing wrong with that at all. There is a reason why the statistics mentioned earlier show that medication is used to treat mental illness in so many people around the world. Whilst medication wasn't my chosen path, it doesn't mean that I don't think it is effective in some cases. If you are using medication and it is working for you the best part is that there is nothing stopping you from using the tools in this book to help you improve your life further. By empowering ourselves with knowledge, tools and strategies, we are doing everything within our control to help ourselves.

If you are using medication it must be used as one part of a holistic strategy. Taking medication does not mean that you can sit back and leave your mental health responsibilities to your prescription alone. Similar to seeing a psychologist, you still need to work and put the effort in at your 'mental gym' to cultivate a long-lasting positive mindset. Whether you use medication for the rest of your life or not is totally up to you. I just want to help you cultivate a positive mindset which may result in even more happiness in the future. If your goal is to reduce your medication dosage in the future, speak with your doctor and if this is right for you, put a plan in place to help reduce your dosage slowly.

Whether you use medication or not, one of the tools that I believe will help you the most in the redesign of your mind is Cognitive Behavioural Therapy (CBT). I practice this by rewriting my thoughts and I will show you how you can do it too. You can practice this on your own or with the help of a psychologist. Studies show that CBT can be at least as effective, if not more effective than antidepressant drug therapy (Burns, 1980). Going back to *Feeling Good: The New Mood Therapy* (1980) by Dr Burns, the first chapter of the book discusses a study where participants were given either antidepressants or CBT, with the results dramatically showing that CBT was more effective in reducing depression than medication. This study reinforces my belief that your thoughts have a significant impact on your emotions. The good news is that even if you have chosen medication as your form of treatment, you can still practice CBT!

There are other things that you can do to help prevent depression. A recent study found that 12% of cases of depression could have been prevented if participants undertook just one hour of physical activity each week. The study also found that people who reported doing no exercise at all were 44% more likely to developing depression when compared to those who exercised one to two hours a week (Blackdoginstitute.org.au, 2019). It is pretty awesome to know that we can dramatically reduce our chances of developing depression just by exercising for at least two hours each week!

Regardless of where you stand on the use of medication, it is up to us to play an active role in our treatment of mental illness. Medication may or may not play a part, but either way it is important to remember that there are other ways to help beat depression. If you choose to use medication, remember to engage the other tools available to help build a holistic wellbeing strategy that gives you the best chance of success.

CHANGE YOUR MINDSET OR CHANGE YOUR ENVIRONMENT?

It is amazing that when going through anxiety or depression, if one event changes for the better, your feelings may snap back into happiness. A common example to demonstrate how this works is a relationship breakup. Have you or someone you know ever broken up with someone and been inconsolable? But not long after they are back with their ex or found someone new, and their life is great again. They 'had' depression and now they don't. The moment that *the event* changed in their life, things went back to normal. In this case it was the person's *environment* that changed (they got back with their ex or found a new partner), and they did not change their *mindset*. What we talked about in early chapters was changing your mindset – which is in your control. Sometimes changing our *environment* is not possible because the other person might not want to get back with us or we can't find someone new right away. Whether a change of environment or a change of mindset is what we need will depend on the situation – but we can always work on our mindset so why not start with that? To bring about lasting change we need to develop a positive mindset to help us get through life's challenging events, particularly if we are unable to change our environment. When I went through my first major depression I tried to deflect the blame and thought that changing my environment would solve all my problems. I blamed my job and thought that quitting my management position would help cure the pain. The support of mentors helped me stay in the role and redesign my mindset instead. Well I didn't really redesign my mindset; all that I did was suppress the negative emotion so that I wouldn't let my mentors down which would turn out to be worse in the long run. The short-term positive was that this led me out of this round of depression; however the negative was that I did not address my mental health and my overconfidence grew. Instead of working on my mindset, I overloaded myself with work and future plans of business success, which ultimately led to a larger bout of anxiety and depression when the new challenges in life presented themselves.

Flash forward to a few years down the track when I had my businesses and felt isolated and on the wrong path, I learnt that I didn't have the right mindset. Yes, I needed to change my environment too, but having a positive mindset would have helped me get through this time with much less self-destruction. After I closed the business and moved into an environment which I much rather enjoyed, I learnt that sooner rather than later, life was going to throw another challenge at me. Sure, I can try to run away from the problem by changing my environment, but I didn't feel that this was going to help me live a happy, healthy life in the long run. I didn't want to leave myself exposed again and it was now time for a complete overhaul of my mind and a rebuild of my thoughts. Eventually I learned that much of our strength in the challenging times comes from our thoughts. Developing courage, grit, determination and a positive mindset is all part of what I needed to work on to get through the tough times that life will no doubt throw at me again. Just like I did all those years ago, I want you to go back and think about what it is that you want to work on first? How are you going to challenge yourself to redesign the way you think? Of course I am going to help you, but you need to cultivate the drive and determination to help you get there.

Depending on your own personal circumstances, you may find that one of either a mindset or environment change may be more challenging. For example changing your environment could be harder for you if you have a family and a big mortgage. Maybe you need to focus on changing your mindset first. Do you know anyone who has just packed up their stuff and left? Maybe someone who has quit their job and booked a random holiday overseas with a week's notice? Maybe someone who decided to move to a new country? This may have even been you at one point in time. Either way the people that make this kind of change are the ones that decided that they needed a change of *environment*. Maybe this is a reason why some people are happier than others – because it is not easy to proactively review your life and actively change direction. It takes a lot of courage. Learning to bring in a willingness to change and an ability to adapt will help put your mental health in a positive state no matter what changes happen to your environment in the future. No longer will we be fixed in our approach to life. We now look forward to constantly redesigning the way we think and the way we behave in the pursuit of our ultimate purpose which is just to be happy.

DOWN BUT NOT OUT

When you are depressed you are down. I know. It is ok to feel down but it is not ok to feel so down that you want to take your own life. Suicide is never a necessary option but unfortunately there are times when people see suicide as the only way out. In 2017 the ABS found that suicide was the 13th leading cause of death in Australia. This is up from 15th place in 2016 (Abs.gov.au, 2019). What is even more horrific is that in 2017 ABS also found that the leading cause of death for Australian people aged 15-44 years was suicide (Abs.gov.au, 2019).It saddens me to think that young people are choosing to end their life. It's not just young people who suffer, with suicide being the second leading cause of death of those aged 45-54 (Abs.gov.au, 2019). Even in our older life, a time when we have already overcome many challenges, we are choosing suicide as a way out. Why are governments and community leaders not doing more about educating and conditioning our people? Governments and companies spend a great amount of money protecting our borders, policing our communities, and maintaining our hospitals – yet they don't spend enough time or money on one of our biggest killers – mental illness. How many young people have tried to take their life but failed? How many stopped at the last minute? How many just go on living with the dark cloud of depression hanging over their heads? The ABS statistics don't give us this information.

We need to understand that depression is not a life sentence. Help is available. By ending our lives by choice at such a young age, we don't even get the opportunity to find out if things were going to get better. Maybe the latter years of our life were going to be the best ones? Samuel L Jackson's first big movie came out when he was in his 40's. Colonel Sanders franchised KFC in his 60's. Charles Darwin, at the age of 50, published *'On the Origin of Species'* which shaped the theory of evolution. These people literally changed the world in one way or another, and yet they never would have known what was possible if they took their own lives in their 20's or 30's. Maybe just like these world changers, the best is yet to come for you? There is only one way to find out – and that is to live on. This is why I am so passionate about mental health and cultivating a positive mindset. Think about how many people we can help just by letting people know that they are not alone and that there are things they can do to beat depression. We need to work together to spread the awareness of mental health and as a collective make a difference. I want everyone to believe that it is ok not to be ok. I want them to understand that they are not alone and have faith that things will get better. Redesigning your mind, and your life, won't happen overnight. It will take a lot of hard work, but it is worth it. Whilst much of the stigma around mental health is dissipating, we still have a long way to go before people understand how important mental health is and that there is always a better action to take instead of suicide.

HELP

Having a desire to help others is something that helped me with my own recovery. Maybe this is something you want to do on your own, and that is totally fine. I found helping others made me feel better about my own problems – whilst also having someone else to support me. The buddy system, looking after each other, is used in many situations because it works. If I had experienced depression 20 years ago things would have been different. The ability to support others and receive support in return would not have been available as depression was not talked about. You just got on with things. Writing this book would never have been a consideration. As a society we have become more open to discussing and sharing our feelings and seeking help but in reality statistics show we still have a long way to go.

If someone is a little overweight they have the opportunity to hire a personal trainer to help them lose some weight. They tell all their friends about it, getting praise for wanting to pursue a healthier body. Instagram posts of their progress are liked by many and they feel great after losing a few kilos. Let's compare that to someone who is mentally overweight and decides to join a 'mental gym' to redesign their mind. The person has the option of engaging a psychologist (personal trainer for the mind) to help them. They put in place coping strategies and different techniques to deal with depression and anxiety. After a period of time they may have made a lot of progress and are now feeling great! Is there any talk with friends and family about this? Is there an Instagram post flashing a big smile and a caption confirming their progress? Do they name and thank their psychologist (personal trainer for the mind) publicly? Of course not! Imagine a world where mental health is just as much a part of life as losing weight. Popular TV shows focused around weight loss and getting fit could be made for mental health as well. We can applaud those that get through the challenge and support those that still need help.

I know we can get there but we still have a long way to go. I have seen firsthand how some people react when you talk about mental health. I have had someone approach me saying *Jenny couldn't cope so she's gone on sick leave depressed, some people are weak*. This ignorant person was unaware that I once suffered from mental illness, and that I once 'couldn't cope'. These people also don't understand that not only are they putting negative energy on to other people, but they are also indirectly putting pressure on themselves, because if they ever experience depression, they will see themselves as being 'weak'. I know what it is like to be the ignorant person too. Before I dealt with my mental illness I couldn't understand what the big deal with mental health was. Now I know all too well that mental illness is real and that we need to support those dealing with these challenges.

I now wear my experience with mental illness as a badge that gives me the opportunity to continuously improve. I want to help other people so that fewer people have to go through what I went through, and no one considers suicide as an option. That said I do know that for others it can be disheartening. If this is you, remember that you don't need to let anyone's thoughts, biases or opinions effect how you feel. They have no idea what you are going through. Maybe one day they will experience their own challenges with mental health – and if this day comes they will finally understand how strong you are. You can help change the world by sharing your stories, your fears, your insecurities, your progress and most of all by supporting those who are having challenges with mental health. This starts by supporting yourself. We will change the world by redesigning one mind at a time.

UNCLE PETE

My uncle Pete was a great guy who was always the life of the party. When I was a kid he would take my brother, my cousin and me down to the park to let off fireworks while the rest of the adults stayed back at the house. He was a hard worker who also liked to enjoy himself. Pete had a 'normal' life with a good job, a wife, a daughter, and a mortgage. He was loved by everyone that knew him. He was well acquainted with life's challenges, including a successful campaign to beat cancer in his 30's. We thought he was indestructible.

All of a sudden we noticed a change in him. He wasn't his usual self. He was now unsettled and full of worry. This was early 2000, a time when we knew less about depression. We just thought that depression was something he would get through. Now I don't know or ever plan to know the full story of what went on in his life. Maybe there was a significant reason why he felt that way and maybe not. But one thing I know is that all the signs that he needed help were there. He needed to redesign his mind but he didn't know how. We didn't know either. He was a solid guy who weighed over 100 kilograms – but all of a sudden he became skinny and his physical appearance started to reflect his state of his mind. One night, unexpectedly we received the worst news.

When my kind, loving Uncle Pete took his life everyone was in shock. Those that knew him couldn't believe it. The friendly, happy guy took his own life and left behind an awesome family and set of friends. The sound of mind, non-depressed Uncle Pete would not have taken this action. He would have joked that he would rather have a beer and watch the football.

When someone takes their own life they not only leave those who love them behind, grieving and hurting, but they rob themselves of the amazing opportunities in life and the chance to be free of depression. It's a weird feeling if you know someone close to you has taken their own life. You immediately feel responsible and as if you should have seen it coming. You feel as though you could have done more to help. I remember Pete asking me to go to a special tour of Adelaide Oval about a year before he died because he had a spare ticket. I was too busy to go and we never got to share that experience. After he died I wished I had gone. I blamed myself for not being a better nephew. *Maybe if I had more fun with him then things would have been different.* Now I know that I cannot blame myself for what happened, but what is in my control is to help myself and others with their mental illness.

Pete was a simple, happy guy who wasn't driven by money, greed or anything else, yet he took his own life. Sometimes I think about what he would say to me if we could talk for a few minutes. I am sure that he would love to go back and change it if he could, but that doesn't matter now anyway. The main thing is that he is at peace and I will do my part to try and save other people from the same fate. The story of my Uncle Pete does not have to be my story, your story, or the story of someone you know. I believe that at the time my uncle didn't want to be a burden to anyone and he thought it would be better for everyone if he wasn't around. But I can tell you that to this day everyone still misses him, and we would give anything to see him again. Never think that you are a burden to anyone. Depression is only a stage of your life. It will get better if you give it time. Whether it is a change of your mindset or your environment, remember that it is up to you.

If you knew that you were going to have ten years of pain, for one year of happiness, would you do it? I know that I want that one year of happiness and it is one of the reasons why I chose to push through dark caves towards the beach of paradise. Some days are spent in the caves, but it is all part of the journey. Maybe if our collective awareness of depression had been different and Uncle Pete had been given the right support, he would have still been here today with his family, still supporting his beloved football team, the Adelaide Crows. I will forever miss the banter we shared when his Adelaide Crows took on my Port Adelaide Power, but maybe his story will help save someone else. Depression is a short-term pain that we never need to treat with a lifetime sentence.

Just like walking through the caves to get to the beach of paradise, there will be days of your journey that are challenging. At times like this it is important to remember that even the most positive, happy person is not 100% happy all of the time; which technically means that they are somewhat de-pressed too. We need to continue to spread the word and grow as a society turning mental health into something cool. We need to use stories like mine, yours and my Uncle Pete's to empower people and help them understand that there is help out there and we will get through this together. We can start by sharing our progress on social media using the hash tag #redesignyourmind. Feel free to tag my Instagram page @wellnesshealth17 to share your journey with like-minded followers.

CHAPTER FOUR
UNDERSTANDING ANXIETY

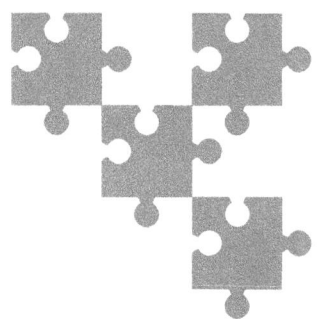

Anxiety is something that everyone has dealt with whether they knew it or not. When you engage in public speaking on the first day of a new job; when you go on a rollercoaster - these are all moments of anxiety. Anxiety is basically the fear of what is about to happen. Some anxiety, like the rollercoaster, can be seen as a fun or 'good' anxiety, whereas most other anxiety causing events are not something that we want to experience. When we experience what we see as bad anxiety our 'flight or fight' response kicks in. We experience physical symptoms such as nausea, tense throat, turning stomach and dizziness. Similar to depression, in a lot of cases anxiety is situational and once the unknown moment has passed everything returns to normal and the anxiety dissipates. A little bit of anxiety for a short period of time is bearable and helps us grow but when it starts to control our lives, being evident without good reason, we need to make changes. This anxiety is known as General Anxiety Disorder (G.A.D.).

Anxiety and depression are like the bash brothers from the Mighty Ducks movies – they love to work together and get up to no good. When one of them shows up to a party, it's not too long before the other one turns up. Telling anxiety or depression to leave, or getting annoyed by their presence, or making a scene, is just going to add fuel to the fire they need to encourage them to stay even longer and have even more of a party. Just like acceptance of an annoying mother-in-law, we need to acknowledge them, accept them, not refuse them entry, and watch them come and go without a care for how long they stay and what they try to do to us in that time.

Fear, stress, being scared, worried, concerned, apprehensive, uneasy, troubled, distressed, edgy, tense, bothered, disturbed are all code words for anxiety. Basically, the fear about what is about to happen next. Buddhism and other practices talk about living in the present and that if you are truly living in the present there is no anxiety – because there is no future, *yet*. If we all lived in the present moment with absolutely no thought about what was next, there would be no anxiety. This is something we can all work on with *mindfulness;*

but the fact is that we can only take it one step at a time, because as humans with conscious minds we *do* think about the future. We make plans, we set up goals, we buy houses with 30-year mortgages, we enrol in 3-year courses, we make commitments, and we get married. No matter how 'in the moment you are', most of us are going to have at least some underlying thought towards the future. We need to redesign our thinking, watering down the pressure these thoughts place on us, so that we can live without constant fear at the back of our minds.

STRESSED OUT

I learnt that stress was a big part of my life when someone found the first grey hair on my head at the age of 24. Whether the grey hair came from stress or not, it is fair to say that I was stressing myself out with my negative thoughts and high expectations. Hopefully the changes I have made over the past few years will stem the flow of grey hairs in the future – or at least I can tell myself that it will! Something as simple as a grey hair is a great example of how we can stress ourselves out. Previously I would worry that more grey hairs would come, and even though it wasn't a big worry, it was something that would increase the pressure and build on my other worries. With my new positive mindset, I am happy with being the next George Clooney.

Stress is just another code word for worry, which really means you are anxious about something. You might be stressed that you are not going to get everything done, or that you have too much going on in life, or that someone is putting pressure on you. Later on, we will work on ways to help find the real reasons why you are stressed, and then either work on changing your mindset or changing your environment.

THE FEAR OF FAILURE

The fear of failure has had a huge influence on my life. I am still learning to cope with it but it is something that we have been conditioned by society to avoid at all costs. How many movies involve a guy who is down and out, who eventually comes back and wins the tournament, or wins the girl, or saves the day? There is usually a happy ending and we all leave the cinema feeling happy and accomplished. We might think that this is how life should be. We are in a society where success is rewarded constantly and effort is all too often only rewarded when it is associated with success. One or many failures do not define who you are. Failure is not permanent. Failure does not need to be negative. Instead failure could be seen as a stepping stone on the path to success. There are some movies that give us hints that failure can be part of success. I know that Star Wars isn't for everyone, but I am going to use the force and mention it anyway. In one of the latest episodes, Luke was dealing with failure and feeling down and out (*yes, even Luke Skywalker, the greatest Jedi Master who ever lived, gets depressed and runs away from his troubles, so why do you need to be so ashamed about your challenges?*), but thankfully Yoda showed up for a timely chat. Yoda gives words of wisdom, emphasising to Luke that 'failure is our greatest teacher'.

Would a hero like Luke Skywalker be considered a failure because he failed at one point in his life or would he be a success because he saved the universe multiple times in the preceding years? What about if a planet with millions of people were blown up due to his error? What if the first planet he tried to save was blown up due to his error? Should Luke give up now and rule himself a failure for the rest of time, or should he take the lessons learnt and use them to help him save the universe as the hero that we know him as? Hopefully it is clear now that ruling ourselves a failure at any point in time is just giving us a negative label that will lead to negative emotions. We fail and we learn. We learn and we grow. I remember when I felt like the biggest failure because I decided to close my business. Was I a 'failure' because I didn't stay in the business forever and that I didn't enjoy it? Or was I a success because I helped many people during this time? Or was this venture a success because it was just one step in the direction of a future success? If you look at the big picture you will find it much easier to remove the pressure of the small 'failures' that everyone in life will endure and better understand that it is all part of your journey towards success.

Imagine if someone created a painting of your life – it might be an awesome beach, a pretty garden, paradise, the New York skyline, maybe all of your family and friends too. Anything you want. I am sure that it would look awesome. But imagine if you only looked at the not so pretty parts – you would think that your life was no good; but this is only one part of the picture. Some parts of the picture are not going to look as nice as others and that is ok, because as a whole it is one pretty cool picture. The best part is that we still have time to design how the rest of it is painted.

DOES IT REALLY MATTER?

Anxiety likes to take over and create an effect of the spinning mind where things just get faster and faster and the anxiety gets larger and larger. One thing I like to ask myself now is 'does it really matter'. Sure, there will be consequences from your actions, but we need to remove the pressure that anxiety is putting on us unnecessarily. Think back to all the times you have stuffed up in your life. Has it resulted in a lifetime of doom and regret? Of course not! Anxiety is a result of our mind telling us that the consequence of what is about to happen will be too much to bear if it goes wrong. However, by asking ourselves *does it really matter*, maybe we can release some of the grip of anxiety. Does it really matter if we turn up to dinner 30 minutes late? Does it really matter if we lose our job? Does it really matter if you break up with your partner? Does it really matter if you embarrass yourself? You can recover from all of these events – many people have and many people will after you too. You won't be broadcast on CNN and shown off to the world – and even if you are, even if it's the most entertaining clip on YouTube, it won't be long before there is something new that takes the spotlight off your hardship. Eventually the world will effortlessly move on, meaning you can move on too.

By learning to take the seriousness out of the situation we can reduce our feelings of anxiety. One of the ways to do this is to have a laugh at ourselves. Without putting yourself down, if you can see the funny side of the situation or try to have a laugh about it, the anxiety will reduce. If laughing doesn't work, you can also ask yourself if you will still be thinking about this issue in a 100 years' time. The question is a mind twister because it is most likely that in 100 years' time you are going to be dead or at a stage of your life where you really wouldn't care about something that happened 100 years ago. If there is going to be a time in the future where it doesn't really matter, then you can ask yourself if it really matters at all. Whether you believe that you will get over the potential consequences of this anxious event in 10 days or 100 years, you might as well not worry about it now and just live your life.

MY ANXIETY

So let's go back to the long list of doctors' appointments I had when I was most anxious. I had dizziness, tingles throughout my body, trouble sleeping, heart palpitations, throbbing in the arm, and even body twitches (yes, I looked like a crazy man). I had constant pressure at the back of my head that would not ease up. It's known as hypertension, where the muscles in the back of your neck which lead up to your head are so tense that you feel like the pressure is going to make your head explode. It's a weird feeling but it was one that I lived with for years. I also found myself in a daze at times with mind-fog clogging up my thought processes. I had reduced concentration, stomach cramps, nausea and troubles with eating. During my first major experience with anxiety, even just looking at food would give me a stomach pain and an instant feeling that I was going to throw up (*if only I hadn't eaten that Chicken on that plane, I would never had caught the stomach bug. Yeah, sure Stef, blame the chicken again…*) As you know, anxiety was the true cause of this ongoing illness. The mind-body connection is unbelievably strong and my body was trying to tell me something.

    I keep referring to movies and here is another one for you. How good is the movie *'Inception'* starring Leo DiCaprio? *I love Leo…*Spoiler alert for those who haven't seen it, but the movie centres on living inside your dreams. The catch is that if you die in your dream, you die in real life too. I like this because it demonstrates (in a fictional way) how powerful the mind and our thoughts are. Even if there is nothing physically wrong with your body, if your mind thinks that there is something wrong, then you will fall victim to all the symptoms and ailments of an illness (or even death). Relating this to the real world, anxiety and depression can have such a grip on your mind that your body feels like something is wrong. When my mental health was at its poorest state my body was reacting as if it were truly sick. Headaches, skin rashes, poor digestion, fatigue and dizziness are just a few ailments to mention. My body was listening to the mind and thought that I was physically sick. I ignored the symptoms for too long as I never believed that these bodily symptoms were a result of anxiety, depression and stress. Once my mind got better the ailments went away just as quickly as they had come!

    Maybe you are still at the stage where you don't believe that these symptoms are a result of your anxiety or depression? I went through blood tests, stomach tests, specialists, trips back to the doctor, and I think I nearly crashed the Google server with the amount of diseases I would look up within a day. This was only fuel for the anxiety fire. Maybe you are adding fuel to your own fire of anxiety? Maybe it is time to accept anxiety and get to work on redesigning your life. I know that it is not easy to think about but if we want to get better we need to acknowledge and accept these things. It is time to accept and tell yourself that you are not sick with an unknown jungle disease that the doctors cannot identify. They have identified your dis-ease and it is called anxiety. What we need to do, is have true acceptance of our anxious emotions. Another great read that helps with accepting anxiety is *Feel the fear and Do It Anyway* – by Susan Jeffers. Susan talks about tackling the symptoms head on and accepting them as part of the giant ride of life. You acknowledge the fear but still do it anyway! This was HUGE for me! It changed how I saw anxiety – it became something that would probably always be there, but who gives a shit; I am going to live my life anyway. Funnily enough when you say this, often the anxiety decreases! If you feel the symptoms of anxiety coming on and you think that you are about to have a panic attack, learn to accept the panic attack. You immediately remove the power of the panic attack because you have decided to let it happen. You are no longer a victim who has a panic attack pushed on to them; you are accepting the panic attack into your life. Tell yourself, *Oh, here comes another panic attack. Its ok I have had one of these before. It will only last a few minutes anyway. I am not going to fight it. I am just going to observe.* This is just an example and you can make your own self-talk that works for you, but the point is that we are taking the power away from the panic attack. We are removing the severity by not fighting it, and whilst it sounds counterintuitive, the more you practice this, the less likely a panic attack will come, and if it does, the less likely it is going to be severe. Your *fear* of the panic attack is now gone.

There were times where I really wanted to escape the physical symptoms of my mental illness. This just made things worse. Counter intuitively, the first step to making the symptoms go away was to accept them. This involved rewriting my thoughts until I truly didn't care about them. *Stef, you are still able to function as well as you could before; you have had every medical test in the book and no physical illness has been found; no one can see, hear or smell the symptoms; so does it really matter? Not really!* After my acceptance of the symptoms, amazingly the symptoms faded away! I had symptoms for nearly two years and was excited to see that they were gone! Unfortunately, the symptoms came back because I noticed that they were gone, giving them back power. I pulled myself back into line and told myself that I needed to accept the symptoms whether they come or go – which gave me the power back, removing the symptoms once again. I no longer fear the symptoms and allow them to come and go as they please. They don't come along often, but when they do I use them as a tool, an alert system, that is telling me there is something that I need to address in my life. Using these symptoms to my advantage has turned something I fear into something I love!

    We need to work on the reason why you feel anxious. Is it because you are scared of what people think about you? That you are being judged? That people see you as a failure? By finding out the real reasons why you are anxious you can then work on cultivating the right mindset to beat it. No I am not anxiety free and I don't just wave my magic wand when anxiety arrives; but now I can better acknowledge when I am feeling anxious and accept it, using the right tools to help the anxiety on its way. We cannot seek to avoid anxiety, because that will make us anxious by trying to avoid it. Whether you need to change your environment (a new job, a new partner, a new city) or change your mindset (new thought processes and behaviours); you will need to acknowledge the anxiety, accept the anxiety and then do something about the anxiety – which we will now get started on.

CHAPTER FIVE
WHO GIVES A F*CK

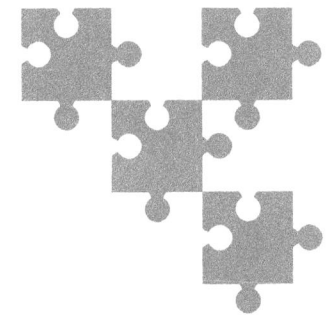

*The Subtle Art of Not Giving a F*ck* by Mark Manson (2016) is an inspirational book that has a few methods that we could all apply to our lives, with the general premise being that we need to give less of a f*ck. However, whilst not giving a f*ck can really help with living a happy life, unfortunately for me, *I still give a f*ck*. I've tried not giving a f*ck, but it's not for me. I mean if you really didn't give a f*ck any more then you wouldn't need to read another book. I am guessing that just like me you may still give a f*ck. Yes, we need to give *less* of a f*ck about certain things, but we can still give a f*ck. Do you give a f*ck about your family, your wellbeing or your health? Of course you do! How about we don't give a f*ck about what doesn't matter and start spending more time on what we do give a f*ck about.

I have learned to better identify whether I give a f*ck about something or not. If the boss says that I am not trying hard enough at work and need to lift my game, is this actually something I give a f*ck about? I might tell myself that I am trying my best – and they can fire me if they expect more than I am capable of. I can also take notice of what my boss tells me and consider that they may be right. I then have to decide whether I want to lift my game, or f*ck off and do something else (*man, you are really loving the word f*ck in this chapter*). What the boss says is not what matters. What does matter is what is important to me and whether this job fits in with where I want to be in life.

In the past, feedback like this would have put me into defensive mode and I would fire back. Now I know that I have the power to take that statement however I see fit and redesign the way I feel about it (by using the right thought processes). We must only give a f*ck about things that really matter. Your boss and your job can have a massive effect on how you feel as a person. If you feel inside that this is not the right place for you, or that you are being pressured or bullied into doing work that you really don't give a f*ck about, then pack up your stuff and leave. As you will learn in this book, forget about the money or the career that you are leaving behind – if it doesn't make you happy inside all it is going to do is waste your positive energy on something negative. Next time something happens and you are ready to fly off, you can think to yourself, *Do I actually give a f*ck about this?* Do I want to allow my happiness to be affected by something that I might not even remember in a few weeks' time? Is there another job or pursuit I can take on in my life? It's time to stop giving a f*ck about the things that don't matter.

REDESIGNING WHAT YOU GIVE A F*CK ABOUT

What do you give a f*ck about? Write them down. It could be things like fun, family, friends, new experiences, career, spending time at the beach or a hobby. Write down 4 or 5 groups of things that you absolutely give a f*ck about. This is all you ever need to give a f*ck about. Everything else in life *really doesn't matter.*

Did you write down that you give a f*ck about 'what everyone else thinks'? If you did then we have a lot of work to do; if you didn't, then why the f*ck do you put such an emphasis on how many likes you get on Facebook, what people say about you, what people don't say about you, how we look and how big your house is compared to your friends? It's time to redefine what is important and leave all the false wants behind. Writing down the values/qualities/things that you truly care about puts them out there to the universe, giving them importance as you travel your journey. If you wrote down that family is the number one thing to you, and your career was fifth, does this mean that putting in ten hours of overtime a week for a few extra dollars is actually worth it? Does it mean that you can now give up chasing a career that may lead to more dollars and less happiness? What would your family advise you to do? Have you ever thought about asking them what they want you to do? If your family is the thing that you give a f*ck about the most, why don't you ask them. *'Hey Lisa, would you and the kids rather I stay back at work each day to earn extra money so we can go to Thailand at the end of the year; or would you rather have me at home having fun with the kids every night?'* There is no right or wrong answer. Some families will want the holiday and others will not give a f*ck about it.

Do you have people that let you down because you give a massive f*ck about them and they do not give a f*ck about you? We have all been there. Unfortunately, you may be in a category that is lower on their rank of things that they care about, or maybe not even on the list at all. A younger version of myself would say, *'Well, that's it, I am not going to try anymore, and I don't care about them'*, but that's not going to bring happiness either. What we need to do is accept that they may not care about us on the same level as we care about them. What is important is that we care about them on a level that brings us happiness, accepting that they will not return the care on the same level. If you are not happy with this arrangement then maybe it is time to move, putting your effort elsewhere.

REDESIGNING YOURSELF

So, we have established what we don't give a f*ck about and what we do give a f*ck about. We can now use this to change where we spend our energy. First, we need to realise that we cannot change others. This is not 'Redesign Your Partner's Mind'. How many people are in a relationship with someone that they are *hoping* will change? Unfortunately, *you cannot change anyone*. You can certainly *influence* people, but *you* cannot change them. Only they can decide if they want to change and we must accept that we can only redesign our own lives.

Expecting someone to act on your requests or influences will only leave you disappointed. The moment you accept that the only change you can make is the one within yourself, the more accepting you will be of others and their decisions, and the more loving and happier you will be. You can lead a horse to water, but you can't make it drink. If you try and pull the horse's head down to the water, it might take a drink, it might not, but again it's not up to you. The horse has to want to drink before it will drink. *Yeah, Stef loves analogies.*

Upon reflection of my younger years – I knew what was important to me, with my top five things being family, relationships, friends, financial stability, fun, and health (mental and physical); however, I did not know how to *balance* these five things. Financial stability was always top of the list, but it was only my insecurity that led me to believe I needed this to help make my other areas such as family, friends, fun and health succeed. I thought that if I took care of the financial stability first and put all of my effort there, the other four things would take care of themselves. Unfortunately, this wasn't the case. How many people do we know that have money and a big house but end up getting divorced because they are never home? We need to truly believe that money, fame or riches do not buy happiness. Below is how I saw the world, thinking that financial success was my main goal, (and I don't blame myself for feeling this way after falling for society's lure to money and fame). Further below is how I try to live my life now. I am not perfect but the balance is so much better than what it was. Work out how much time and energy you want to spend in each of your chosen areas – and remember that nothing is forever. Things can and will always change.

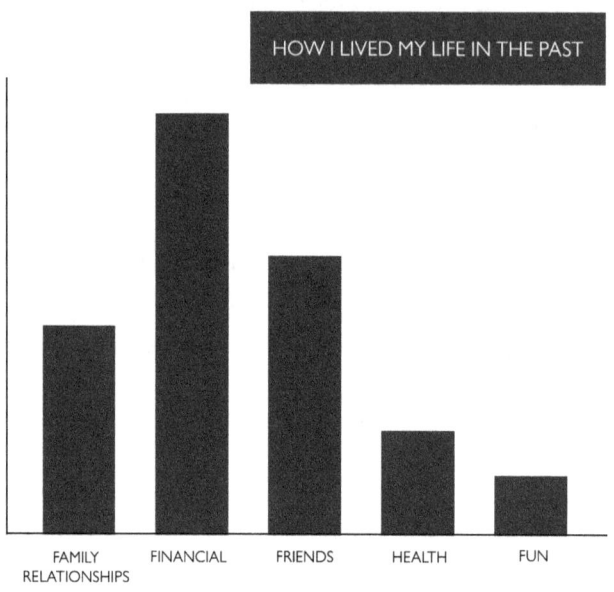

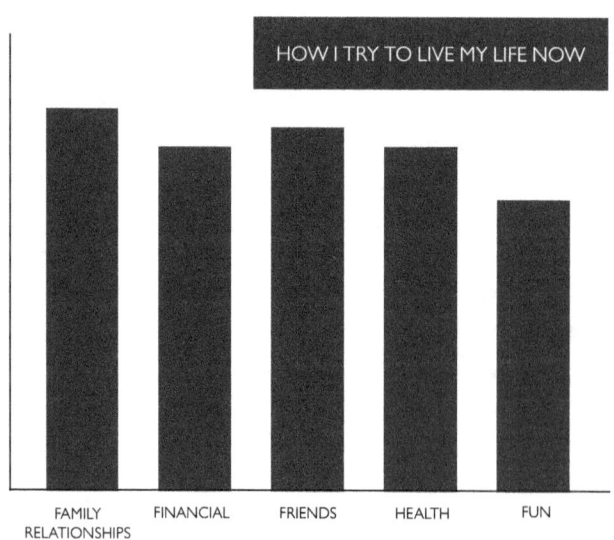

Things will get out of balance from time to time, but this is part of the enjoyment of life. With awareness and understanding we can make adjustments when required. If you have a big deadline at work, you might spend more time on the financial part of your life, but it's important to make sure this is temporary and doesn't put you permanently out of balance. Yes, when you get a new partner and love is in the air –sure your relationship might take over but we need to keep in touch with our friends, our physical health (*I'm guessing that will be active with a new partner*) and most importantly we need to maintain the balance. Has someone you know ever started a new relationship and dropped every other hobby or interest or friend in their life? What happens when the relationship ends? Depression often hits because they have put all of their eggs of happiness in the one basket. Yes, things will get out of balance from time to time, but no matter how good the sex is, keep the balance because you never know when it's all going to end!

After drawing your 'ideal world' of happiness, adding how much time and energy you want to spend in each area of importance, you may like to draw a weekly or monthly graph to track how you are going with keeping the balance in your life. This week my graph looks like the one below:

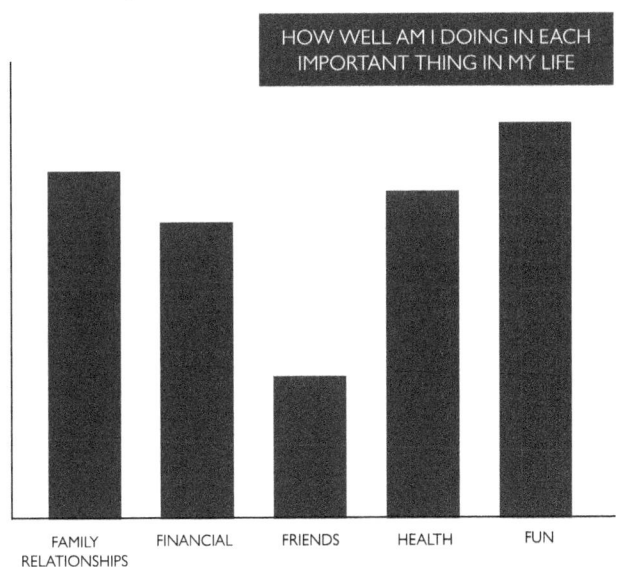

You might be doing really well with 'fun' but maybe you haven't spent much time with your friends lately. This self-awareness will help you to make the adjustment to bring it back into balance. After a while you won't even need the graph and you can just tell when you need to adjust. Another thing that I like about this graph is that it will help you acknowledge that sometimes one area will be up and sometimes one area will be down. Since I have been tracking my life – there has not been one moment where I have had all five things perfect and flying high. So does this mean I remain unhappy and hold off my happiness until it is all perfect? Of course not! My life isn't perfect yet I am the happiest I have ever been! This helps us look at life's big picture and understand that not everything is perfect. We can choose whether to focus on the negatives which will bring about anxiety or depression, or we can focus on the positives which will bring about gratitude and happiness.

CHAPTER SIX
HOW TO REDESIGN YOUR MIND

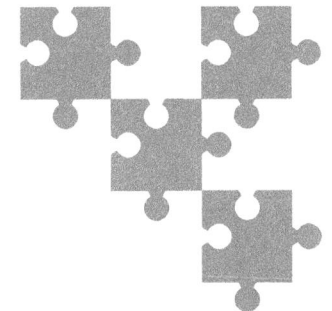

As I mentioned earlier in this book, the first part of my life was relatively easy. I was brought up in your standard Western-upper-middle-class family. Life was pretty free-flowing and up until my early 20's I kicked goals in everything I did. Life was great and I was full of confidence. It wasn't until that dodgy chicken on the plane to the USA (anxiety) that I finally started to understand that life was not always a walk in the park and that anxiety and depression can have a massive impact on your life. The mind-body connection was so powerful that I just didn't believe it. *I must have been sick. How was anxiety causing my body to react this way? Surely my mind was stronger than this.* Well yes, that's the whole point, your mind is strong and if you don't listen to your mind then your body will tell you that something is wrong. And that's what happened. With no awareness, understanding or acceptance of anxiety, my thoughts gave my body and soul a pounding that practically lasted on and off for the most part of four years. Do we really need to feel like this? We live in a time where so many things can bring us happiness, so why do we need to put these unnecessary depressive or anxious states of mind on ourselves? It is time to change the way we think.

Just like I did on my third day of taking anti-depressants, it is time for you to draw a line in the sand and say that enough is enough. It is now time for you to implement the positive behaviours and thoughts that are ultimately going to lead to positive emotions of happiness, gratitude, love and peace. You are now responsible for your happiness; not what happens to you, not what happens to someone else, not what someone else says about you; only you will be responsible for your happiness. Whether the events that happen in your life are fair or not, good or bad, fruitful or debilitating, you will decide your own happiness by empowering your mind with the right thoughts.

Plugging in and empowering the right thoughts are what is going to lead to positive emotions. We are not going to try and push out the negative thoughts, totally the opposite. We are just going to let them float by and we are going to input the thoughts that we want and deserve. Remember that *what fires the brain, wires the brain;* and by firing up new thought patterns, eventually these thoughts will wire your brain, instilling a new positive mindset. Change is the only constant in life. You have been changing your whole life anyway, so you might as well embrace the change and build a mindset and a lifestyle that works for who you want to be. Your new thoughts will eventually deplete anxious and depressive emotions as you disengage thoughts about any negative past by staying in the present, also by not fixating on the future that may or may not happen. If your past wasn't something to be grateful about then you can be grateful that it is over. Your past is in the past. Leave it there forever. Don't live your life dwelling about something that happened to you 5 years ago, 5 months ago, 5 weeks ago, 5 days ago, or even 5 minutes ago. What does this achieve? Similarly with anxiety – do you want to spend your life running through scenarios that may happen in 5 years, 5 months, 5 weeks, 5 days or even 5 minutes' time? This doesn't mean that we don't plan for the future but it means that we remove expectations and concerns about whether something happens or not.

Yeah, I put myself through some massive challenges and tough times dealing with anxiety and depression. However, I am grateful that I have experienced it in the past and now I have the *wisdom* to put myself on a path that is leading me to where I want to go. Now I can use these experiences to help me every day for the rest of my life. Yes, it would have been great if I could have just known these things without ever putting myself through tough times – but that is in the past now. I can now be grateful for the silver lining that has *changed* my life for the better. Some of the methods I used for redesigning my mind are not new – but I have tweaked them in a way that worked for me and ultimately may work for you too. Remember that change is all about trial and error; so if something doesn't work for you then try something else.

What might work for you today might not work for you tomorrow. Always keep in the back of your mind that true change is about constantly seeking ways to grow and evolve as a person. Redesign will be constant. If you are 25 years old, single and with few commitments, a change of environment is going to have fewer restrictions when compared to a 40 year old who is married with 3 kids and a mortgage – but who am I to limit what you can and can't change depending on your life circumstances. You decide. I know that sometimes it feels like we *can't* change, as if something is holding us back. But the fact is that if your life is not where you want it to be and you are miserable – well maybe making a change is a better option instead of living the rest of your life saying you *can't;* even if you are that middle aged woman with kids and a mortgage. Sometimes we feel that it is too late to change, or that we have put too much effort into something to just let it go. We need to understand that what may have seemed like the perfect life five years ago might be torture today. It doesn't mean that you need to disregard the life, people or events that are no longer important to you, but it does mean that you can empower yourself to make whatever change it is that you want to make.

REDESIGNING YOUR MIND

Do you think too much? I do, but it is ok now that I have learnt how to use my thinking to help me. Ignorance is said to be bliss however for people like us –the over-thinkers, I don't think there is a way to learn ignorance; meaning we have to find another way to free ourselves from our mind. Our hardware is a high processing super computer. I love the fact that I am a thinker (*with a super computer*). I like to analyse and understand things, considering different possibilities. What we need to redesign are the thoughts that go into our mind (*the apps, programs and software*) – not the amount of thoughts. Understand that you have some of the world's best hardware installed in your mind. You are capable of processing and understanding lots of things; however you haven't been loaded with the right software. Those ignorant (yet blissful) people are never going to have the hardware and storage capacity that your mind holds; the positive for them is that they are loaded with something a lot simpler that keeps things running at a smooth and easy pace. However for us over-thinkers who have many more programs loaded on to our system, our programs cause our CPU (hardware) to strain and suffer (shown through our mind-body connection symptoms). What we need to do is redesign the software. The thoughts that you choose to cultivate are the thoughts that will eventually keep coming back, leading to positive or negative emotions.

The first step to changing your thinking is to free your mind of the ball and chain. This ball and chain that I speak of is the idea that 'we cannot change our thoughts'. This is bullshit. Acknowledge the fact that you can change your thinking and you can have the mindset that you want to have. When someone says, 'Oh that's just how he is and he will never change', they are right. That person will never change if they believe what has been told to them. Confucius once said that 'the man who says he can, and the man who says he cannot are both usually correct'. The person that acknowledges that they can change will be successful in the redesign of their mind. Would you rather live the rest of your life with the thoughts that have been handed down to you, or would you rather create your own thoughts that empower you to live a happier life?

It is time to learn how to use a powerful, practical tool that was imperative in the redesign of my mind. This tool from the book *Feeling Good: The New Mood Therapy* by Dr Burns (1980) will help change your life. Dr Burns is one of the pioneers of Cognitive Behavioural Therapy (CBT) – something that psychologists still use today to help people get their life back on track. Dr Burns explains how many of our thoughts are 'wrong' in that they are *cognitive distortions* where our thoughts are distorted and based on flawed ideals. Our thoughts lead to our emotions and by having flawed thoughts, emotions such as anxiety and depression will follow. Many of these cognitive distortions have been implanted in our mind by friends, family, our education, our life experiences, the media and social cultures over time.

Many of Dr Burns' tools in his book have been successful for many of his patients. I consider myself another success story and hope that you will join me too. My favourite tool from the book involves rewriting your thoughts as a way of weeding out your cognitive distortions. I see cognitive distortions as 'things that we want to remove from our thinking'. This practice of rewriting our thoughts will involve going deep into your mind and it will help you uncover the root causes of your negative emotions. I know it can be challenging, and it will take time and effort. When I first started it took me over an hour each day because my thoughts were so *distorted* – but thanks to this tool I have successfully cultivated a mindset which I am grateful for. I look back at my old notes and laugh at how many of my negative thoughts had no value and often didn't even make sense. We need to learn to challenge these negative thoughts. We need to be the 'judge' in the court house who says, 'Hey *wait a minute, Mr Negative, is this thought actually true?*' By rewriting our thoughts we rationalise the thought and start to train our mind to bring in the rational thought first – or at least learn to challenge the thought. Remember that we are in no way trying to keep the negative thought out or trying to block it. By rewriting our thoughts we are adding a rational thought to counter the irrational cognitive distortion. Our goal is for our mind to replace the negative thoughts with the rational, true thoughts that will lead to happy and rational emotions.

There are lists of cognitive distortions available online and in books such as *Feeling Good and The Worry Cure* by Robert Leahy (2005); but here is a list of some of my favourite cognitive distortions and a redesign to match. Take a photo of this list and come back to it whenever you think that you have a thought that may be *distorted*.

THINGS TO REWRITE FROM YOUR MIND (COGNITIVE DISTORTIONS)
1. Jumping to conclusions: You jump to a negative conclusion without knowing the facts. 'He doesn't like me because he didn't ask me over this weekend.'
Redesign: How do you know? What evidence have you got?
2. Fortune Teller: You predict a future event will have a negative outcome. 'I am going to fail that test.'
Redesign: How do you know that this will happen? What can you do to potentially change this outcome?
3. Magnification: You exaggerate the importance of negative events. 'They didn't invite me to a party and I am never going to speak to them again.'
Redesign: Does it really matter? What are the positives you can build on from this event?
4. Minimisation & Discounting the positives: You shrink the importance of positive events or qualities. 'I haven't achieved anything special; anyone could have done it.'
Redesign: What have you achieved so far? What can you be grateful for? Can you celebrate the positives?
5. 'Should' Statements: You look at the way the world 'should' be. You put guilt on yourself and others by saying that you 'should do something'.
Redesign: You 'could'. You 'might like to'. Delete the word 'should'.
6. 'What if' Statements: You unnecessarily ask yourself 'what if'. What if something goes wrong? What if I fail?
Redesign: What if I succeed? What if I enjoy myself? What if it works out?
7. Mental Filter: You dwell on the negatives. It could have been the perfect day with one little mishap, but that one mishap is all that you care about.
Redesign: I am going to focus on what is right in my life. What were the good parts of the event?
8. Labelling: You label something with a negative situation. 'I am a loser.' 'He is a wanker.'
Redesign: I have lost on this occasion but I have succeeded at many other things in life. He acts like a wanker at times (but is not permanently labelled a wanker).

THINGS TO REWRITE FROM YOUR MIND (COGNITIVE DISTORTIONS)
9. All or nothing thinking: There are no fifty shades of grey with you. It is black or white. It was either a success or a failure. That person is good or bad.
Redesign: Find the grey in life. Nothing is either a total success or total failure. No one is totally good or totally bad.
10. Unfair Comparisons: You are comparing yourself to who did better than you on a particular task and render yourself inferior because you didn't do as well.
Redesign: I did well and I am happy with what I achieved. I can work to improve and do better next time.
11. Entitled Brat: You think that you are more entitled to a good life than others. When things go wrong you can't believe that it has happened to you.
Redesign: Many other people who were smarter than me have failed before me. I cannot expect to be right all the time. I do better than most but it doesn't mean that I am entitled to anything more than the next person.
12. The Blamer: You like to blame your circumstances on someone or something else. 'I am only acting this way because I was cheated on.'
Redesign: I am responsible for my behaviour and my life. My behaviour has been poor but I will address this and improve. Even if someone has wronged me I will learn from it.
13. Living In the Past: You live in the past and cannot get over it.
Redesign: What happened in the past stays in the past. Learn from your mistakes, missed opportunities or from those who wronged you. Use these events to fuel your drive to become better instead of dwelling on what happened.

These cognitive distortions unnecessarily drive us to negative emotions. Knowing these cognitive distortions and when they are occurring in your mind is the first step to redesigning your mind. The second part is rewriting your thoughts with rational responses. This is what we are going to look at now. I have modified the tool from *Feeling Good* by David Burns into something that worked well for me as shown in the below example.

STEPS TO REDESIGN YOUR THOUGHTS

Step 1 – write down the event.

My girlfriend dumped me.

Step 2 – write down your emotions and the percentage that you feel those emotions

Depressed 50%, disappointed 60%, anxious 80%

Step 3 – write down your negative thoughts associated with event

1. I am a loser. 2. No one will ever stay with me. 3. I am ugly…

Step 4 – now write the cognitive distortion from above next to each negative thought.

1. Labelling. 2. Jumping to conclusions. 3. Magnification/ Labelling

Step 5 – Now rationalise each thought with your rational thought

1. She broke up with me, so what. I still have friends and family. Just because someone broke up with me it does not make me a loser. 2. How do I know that no one will ever want to stay with me? Maybe she just wasn't the right girl for me? And maybe I will have more fun being single anyway. 3. I have picked up girls before, so I must not be that ugly; and some girls like ugly guys anyway.

NOTE – go into as much or little detail as you like on this one. Sometimes I would write a whole page on 'why I am not a loser'. *Sad I know.* But it works. This is a great way to counsel yourself and make yourself feel better.

Step 6 – Now write down your emotions from step 2 (without looking at the %) and then write down the NEW % of the emotion.

Depressed 30%, disappointed 25%, anxious 50%

You will find that most of those negative percentages have come down, which is already a positive and makes you feel great. I am yet to have a time when my negative emotions haven't come down from the original score. Even if it only feels 5% less than what it was when you started writing, then that is a massive win and it empowers you to understand that time will heal this wound, and by using the right thoughts it will heal even quicker.

Step 7 – BONUS STEP FROM STEF– I now write down the positive thoughts and % that I am feeling as a result of rewriting my thoughts.

Happy 40%, ready for change 50% (that's not really an emotion but you know what I mean), grateful 60%.

Writing out the positive emotions at the end makes a massive difference, even if they are the smallest percentage. This last step is something that I adapted into my rewriting of thoughts and I hope that if the author of *Feeling Good* or *The Worry Cure* ever read my book that they would be happy with my continuation of their techniques. I found that adding this step forced me to search for positive emotions and thoughts within my mind. Stretching to think about these positive emotions helped my mind automatically search for them again in subsequent situations. Another reason why I have added step 7 is because often our mind only remembers the last thing that is said in a particular conversation or experience. So, by adding a final step which is a positive, this then leaves you… feeling good! It's just like when you're watching a movie and it finishes with a happy ending. Movie producers spend a great amount of time studying what makes us happy and there is no coincidence why most movies have a happy ending. No matter how challenging the experience for the characters was, because it ended well you walk out happy. You can also adapt this to your conversations with friends, your time at work, or even your day. Something as simple as adding 'have a top day' or 'see you later legend' and putting a smile on your face as you say it makes a massive difference to someone's day and their experience with you. This simple yet effective tool, practised day in, day out will help you successfully redesign your mind. This practice saved my life and helped me on my journey from negative to positive. It will help you too if you believe and give it a good shot. You could even work with a psychologist as your 'personal trainer for the mind' guiding you along the way. If you want to do it on your own, you will need to be committed to practicing daily, but if you believe you can do it then so do I!

DID I CHANGE?

I will admit that redesigning my mind did take time and it will require regular maintenance, especially when challenging events are thrown upon us. The first thing that I noticed after a few weeks of re-writing my thoughts was that I was starting to automatically rationalise the negative thought as it was coming into my head. This was an amazing feeling of progress and it gave me the confidence that lasting change was possible. It's just like exercising your body at a gym. If you train regularly you will start to see *change* relatively quickly. If you go sporadically whenever you feel like it – then you are not going to see any change and ultimately you will give up because you think that it's not working; when in fact it is you that is not working – not working hard enough! Are you going to change your mindset and give something a red hot go or are you going to do it when you feel like it? There's no doubt that you'll have to make sacrifices, mainly to your time, but it will be worth it. I am not a motivator and

I don't plan to motivate you in any way. I am here to inspire you to redesign your mind. If you feel the inspiration and want to do it, then you won't need to be motivated by me or anyone else. You can do it if you commit to rewriting your thoughts and practice it day in, day out. Even if it is just 10 minutes in the morning and 10 minutes at night, it will make a difference.

Start rewriting your thoughts today and in a month's time who knows what your thoughts will be. I found that this one technique of re-writing my thoughts, which is the foundation of CBT, really helped me redesign my mind which was reflected in my emotions. Just make sure whatever it is that you try, you give it a go for at least 21 days to give your mind a chance to adjust and see if you are happy with the results. If it doesn't work, then *change* your game plan and try something else.

As time went on I started to notice the cognitive distortions that were present in other people around me. This was a massive trap that I had to navigate through. Often when we are talking with friends or family, at work, or watching something on TV we come across other people's cognitive distortions. They may say something about a particular situation, or about you, or someone else that you realise is a cognitive distortion. You now have the power to question whether what they say is valid or not. I found that as I got better and better with my thoughts, surprisingly not everyone liked it. I actually had someone say that they didn't like my positive attitude during a challenging situation. How bizarre is that? Unfortunately, not everyone wants to cultivate a positive mindset, and that's ok. *Ignorance is bliss.* It is their choice whether they join us on our journey or not. It wasn't long before I learnt that walking into a room and giving out inspirational, positive comments and talking about how we retrained our mind is not something that everyone wants to hear. Often it makes them feel guilty about the fact that they are still stuck in the old world of thought. We need to understand that not all people have the desire or even the need for change. Our happiness doesn't depend on someone else validating the changes we have made in our life. Our happiness comes from within. This is another reason why I decided to put my story into a book so that people can *choose* to read it if they are seeking help with their mental health.

It is up to you, and only you to redesign your thought processes. Yes, you will have to become more self-aware; yes, it will be a challenge, but yes, it will be worth it. I sometimes wonder what would have happened on my USA holiday if I hadn't had that spell of anxiety. Maybe I would have had the time of my life and decided to spend the next 10 years of my life travelling. Maybe if I had completed the redesign of my mind while I had the business I would have been able to deal with more of the challenges and kept the business ongoing. These are thoughts that I now let pass as things that I will never know the answer to. We will never know which way is right or wrong in life, and that is what makes it so exciting. There is no point running through the playbook of your last relationship and what could have or should have happened. All this will do is lead to negative emotions. We can think back and reflect for a few moments if we choose to; but we need to learn from our mistakes and make the changes that we want to make for the next relationship.

REDESIGN YOUR LANGUAGE

No, I am not talking about learning to speak French, what I mean is that we need to change the way we speak – to ourselves and others. The way you speak has a direct effect on your thoughts and ultimately your emotions. This includes your mannerisms, your body language, and what you *really mean* by what you are saying. Were you really joking when you made a comment about a friend? We also need to understand that what someone hears and what we meant to say may be two different things. Have you ever said something that was taken the wrong way? Have you heard the 2018 craze about the 'Yanny or Laurel' audio? I cannot figure out how anyone in the world hears 'Laurel', but either way this is a great insight as to how we can totally misunderstand what someone else says. How we speak can definitely effect what message we are trying to get across and how it is received by the other person and we need to apply the cognitive distortions principles to our language. The more you practice it, the better it will work. Let's compare the following;

Event: You missed out on a promotion at work

Thought: I'm not good enough, I should have got the job, that other guy is no good for the job, this is bullshit (negative)

Emotion: Pissed off, angry, disappointed, depressed, undervalued, sad.

Compare that to the below;

Event: You missed out on a promotion at work

Thought: I went pretty far and almost got the job. Now wasn't the right time for me but I learnt a lot and now I know what I need to do to get the promotion. The other good thing is that I won't have to bust my ass and stay back to get all this extra work done and I can spend more time having more fun (positive)

Emotion: Acceptance, happiness, gratitude, reflective, ready to set goals, understanding, creative (yes, these aren't all emotions per se but this is how you feel)

The same event resulted in a totally different outcome to your emotions just by changing your thoughts. Yes, I still have negative thoughts popping into my head every day. The difference is that now I let these thoughts float by without ruminating on them. I cultivate the positive thoughts that will help me move forward and get through the challenging events, and you can too if you take the time to rewrite your thoughts.

WATCH YOUR LANGUAGE

The previous scenario is a great example of how just changing a few sentences can make the resulting emotions seem so different. Part of changing our language means also restricting and limiting the usage of words that do not help us, using more of the positive language. Throw away words such as tough, sucked, harsh, disappointing, hard, not easy, difficult, tiring, problem, issue, boring and replace these words with *challenge*. When you have a challenge, this empowers your mind to think of a way it can be overcome, turning it into something that is to be achieved. When you say something is 'hard', this makes you feel like it really is too difficult.

Negative language deflates you and puts you down without you even knowing. Switching to more positive words is a small simple change that works with every sentence. Maybe you and your partner are *going through a tough time*? This doesn't sound too good does it? How does it make you feel if you say it again and again? Not very good, hey? Compare it to saying *my partner and I are having some challenges*. It sounds a lot better doesn't it? It becomes something you can overcome. Your relationship is no longer tough, it is just experiencing a challenge that you can overcome.

Just like the craze with the Yanny and Laurel audio of 2018, the tone and language of what we are saying can be totally misunderstood (or understood) by ourselves and those we are speaking to. Understand that the pitch, tone and timing of what we say has a direct influence on the outcome of how our message is received.

Throughout the journey of redesigning my mind, I learnt to become more in touch with and accepting of my emotions. As I became more aware of my emotions I was able to express them better. I learnt that my subconscious is listening all of the time and whatever I said or thought would be taken in like a sponge. By changing our language we assist the rewiring of our brain because our brain is taking note of what was said last time. How you feel today has a lot to do with what you said, did and thought the day before. As a result this further enhances the idea of creating positive habits and giving ourselves time for change. By redesigning your mind today, you might see the positive results compound over the weeks, months and years of your life.

Your body language, posture, mannerisms, enthusiasm in your speech and confidence in your voice are all important to your mental health. The mind-body connection is way stronger than we think. Have you ever noticed that within a few minutes of chatting to a new person you can tell if they are low in confidence? They didn't actually say 'I have no confidence' – but their choice of words, voice and body language gave it away. Compare this to someone who stands up tall with a confident choice of words and loud voice. Their body language oozes confidence.

Our mind takes note of our body language. It understands our posture, speech and everything else – using them to gauge if we are anxious, depressed or lacking in confidence. If you don't believe me, give it a try. Head to work with a hunched back, no smile, a low voice, lower your head and don't stand up tall. See how you feel. Now the next day go out and stand up tall, smile, and speak with a confident voice. See how you feel. It will actually amaze you how your emotions will change. I still need to remind myself some days to keep this up because it can fall away – because our body language is often something we are not conscious of; but it's just like exercising at the gym – we need to practice regularly to maintain our mental health fitness.

The English word 'anxiety' is derived from the German, Latin and Greek verbs that describe things such as 'to strangle, to squeeze tightly', 'tightness', and 'choking in the throat'. These are all things to do with the body. Why is it that we are using bodily symptoms to explain something known as a problem with the mind? This is because of the unbelievably strong mind-body connection. Sometimes it can be a challenge to know which one is leading the other. Does the body feel tight and stressed because of the mind? Most likely; although it is possible that your mind can become tired and stressed because of a tight or stressed body. In this day and age anxiety doesn't come from chasing lions or trying to find enough food, it relates to many of the challenges we create in our own minds that we need to learn to release ourselves from.

YOU SHOULD CHANGE

I use to love the word 'should'. Looking back to the section on our cognitive distortions, the word should is something that you may want to consider removing from your vocabulary. Saying to ourselves (or someone else) that you 'should' do something is going to create pressure on the mind and emotions of guilt. I was one of the worst at using the 'should' guilt trip on myself. It's the same when you say it to someone else or if someone says it to you. Even with no malice this word still has the same negative effect. You might say to someone (or vice versa), 'You should come out on Saturday night'. This now instantly makes that person feel obliged to come out on Saturday night. If they are unsure of whether they want to come out on Saturday night, they instantly feel like they are going to let you down if they don't. If we say 'I should go to the gym', this instantly puts the pressure on us to go to gym. If we make it to the gym we will feel like a success; if we don't go to the gym our emotions of guilt will follow.

Throw out the word 'should' and replace it with 'could' or 'I would like to', or 'you might like to'. By saying 'we could' or 'I could' or 'you could' in place of 'should', this removes the pressure and empowers us to make a decision. If you choose not to, then there are no negative feelings of guilt, and if you do choose to do it you then feel empowered because you feel as if you made the decision without a forced hand. Saying to someone else 'you should help me clean the house' compared to 'you could help me clean the house' may receive a different response. This subtle change in language can have seriously positive effects.

Often we say things about other people, like 'Sarah should have invited me to that party' or 'my partner should have known better' or 'my boss should have known that I wanted that promotion'. The fact is that this is all a load of crap and all it does is create great expectations for ourselves. Do people always do the right thing? No. Do people always do what is best for you? Why *should* they? I used to (and still sometimes do) feel jealous about the way some things would turn out. *You know, because I worked really hard and I 'should' be really successful.* I saw others who didn't put in the same effort as me but were doing better than me. *This isn't fair. Why wasn't I enjoying the same level of success as them? Things should be different.* No they aren't different and all you are doing is making yourself feel depressed for no reason. I used to think that people 'should' return favours – just like when you go to a bar and buy a round of drinks, and there is that one person who loves to sneak off just before it is their round; they *should* buy the next round of drinks, but they don't. What about that person that you're always there for but they are never there for you? They 'should' have been there! Unfortunately, the answer is *no, no they shouldn't*. We must remove the expectation that if we do something, we will get something in return. If you want to buy your mates a drink, or be there for someone that's important to you, then you do it because you want to help them, or have a drink together, not because you want things to be even and expect them be there for you when you need it.

Removing the word 'should' as often as possible has helped me remove the pressure on my past and future actions. There are times when I 'should' have gone to see someone, or I 'should' have cleaned up; however because I redesigned my language, I did what I felt like doing and what I felt was right for me at the time, without the emotions of guilt. Unfortunately many others will still be stuck in the world of should; which can feel demanding on yourself when they put this language onto you; but we need to stick to what we know is right for us and our own happiness. If you explain the reasons why you did or didn't do something, I'm sure that person will come to understand; and if they don't, well then maybe you *should* reconsider what their opinion means to you. Ultimately you should, I mean could, remove the word should from your language.

THIS TIME NEXT WEEK

I look back now and laugh at how many times I would get dramatically worked up, pissed off, or sad about an event in my life only to find a week later I had new 'challenges' (*not problems*) to replace them. Whatever it was that I was stressing about last week had absolutely no relevance in my life anymore. This was an absolute waste of energy and all it does is keep us in our never-ending depressive, anxious, pissed off or disappointed state. The thing is that there are always going to be new challenges presenting themselves, so you're always going to be in this state unless you rebuild your thought processes. Just like we learnt in the 'When are you going to be happy' section of this book, we cannot wait for all things to be perfectly in line and balanced for us to be happy. So why are you going to spend the rest of your life waiting for things to be perfect? Instead you can enjoy other pursuits in the meantime. One thing that has helped me with my happiness is asking myself, 'Will this matter this time next week?' Whenever I am in the heat of the moment and something is rattling my cage, I ask myself this question. Maybe you can choose to wait until the end of next week before you decide if this is something major or not? By shelving the thought for a week you might find that in many cases it will never be taken back off the shelf because something else will come up in that time.

A little game I play with myself when something pisses me off or gets me feeling down, is to say, 'Ok Stef, let's make a bet. How long is this going to keep you pissed off / depressed or sad for?' *Hmm maybe five days?* Ha! Ok well if you know that you will be fine in five days, then why don't you just get over this now and save your energy? You know that you'll get over it so there's no point wasting the next five days of positive energy on this. This instantly puts a timeline on how long you are going to feel shit about something for. Instantly my mind now feels empowered that I know that I will get over it and I can start to move forward with my life.

As time goes on, maybe that evening or the next morning, I will ask myself if it is still bothering me. *Yep, it's still bothering me.* Ok it is time to rewrite my thoughts, see what cognitive distortions are present and work through this challenge. This discussion with your own mind works wonders. It questions your negative thoughts, it makes you rationalise with your mind and it removes the power of something ruminating again and again. By rewriting our thoughts we can objectively see the cognitive distortions in our thoughts and learn to replace them with thoughts that will better serve our mental health. It will take time though and it will be challenging at first as you may find that there is more work to do on your mind than you first thought – well that's what I found anyway!

So where will you be this time next week? Will you have one week of experience of rewriting your thoughts? Or will you be waiting for a better time to get started? Choosing to delay your start date for any reason could be a thought that you may want to rewrite.

CHAPTER SEVEN
GREAT EXPECTATIONS

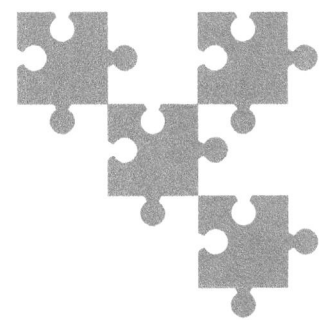

REDEFINING SUCCESS

All of my life I have been ambitious. I have always had the passion, determination and desire for success. For a while things were going well and I could see that my ambition was materialising into material success. I wanted more. More success and more ambition. During the darkest stages of my anxiety and depression, I realised material and financial success was all a load of shit. It is not success; it is *greed*. Some of you may already know this, but for others like me we need to explicitly be told. Jim Carey once said 'I think everybody should get rich and famous and do everything they ever dreamed of so they can see that it's not the answer.' I would have laughed at this when I was younger but now I understand. The problem lies not in our definition of ambition, but in our definition of success.

What does success and ambition mean to you? Does success revolve around what others think of you, your material possessions, the size of your house, how many likes you get on Instagram or being better than someone else? Previously all of these outside influences were so important to me. My ambition was to *be the best* in everything I could be. I now look back at my darkest times of anxiety and depression and am grateful for this experience. If it wasn't for things not going according to plan, who knows what kind of *ambitious, successful,* financial king-pin dick I would have turned out to be. I would have had material success but I am not sure if I would have had the lasting success of love for my family and friends and a passion to live a happy and balanced life.

I cared what people thought of me so much that I thought I needed to be 'successful' to be a valued or wanted person. This again was society playing its part on me, and I accept full responsibility for letting my values be manipulated by society's demands.

Not long after I remodelled my mind and was ready for dating again, I found myself updating my Tinder profile. I was searching for a few words that best described me as a person when I remembered that one of my old words was 'ambitious'. A word I felt I was no longer worthy of because I was no longer dedicating my life to chasing success. This brought me down and left me at a loss as to what to replace it with. If I no longer was ambitious, what was I? Then it clicked. I was still ambitious! In fact I was more ambitious than ever. I was just no longer chasing *material* success. I redefined my definition of success! Being ambitious no longer meant that I had to strive for success in the form of the best job, or the highest salary, or a big house, car, riches or fame. Being ambitious still meant that I still wanted success – but my definition of success would now come in the form of happiness. If I am happy in whatever it is I am doing in life, wherever I am, then I am successful. My ambition is now derived in the pursuit of happiness. That was it. I am now ambitious for happiness. 'Ambitious' was once again the best word to describe me but for totally different reasons! It felt great to jump back on Tinder and add the word 'ambitious' back to the top of the list of words to best describe me.

To be happy I understand that I need to be successful in the areas of my life that are important to me; friends, family, fun, career, financial stability, new experiences – not just sitting on top of the corporate ladder with a Ferrari in the garage. I am now ambitious to seek a balance in all of these areas and be the best person I can be for myself – not for someone else. Not for a flashy Instagram account or what society wants me to be. Isn't it funny that I am now more ambitious than I was before my battle with mental illness? Maybe you will become more ambitious when you find a meaning of success that works for you.

What did success and ambition mean to you before you read the above paragraph? Were you focused on material success? Things you could possess, or say you've achieved? Or was it more emotional, loving, social success? Something that when you sit on your death bed you can say you were glad that you got to experience. If you are still not sure - do you think that anyone lies on their death bed and says, 'Wow, I am so happy that I won that award for being the top salesman for 2018?' Or do you think people will be grateful for the people they met, the experiences they had and hopefully a family that loves them? You know the answer. How much money, fame or riches do you need to have love for yourself and others? Not much (if any). This does not mean we cannot pursue material success. What it does mean is that we can change *our definition* of success and therefore our ambition. We can still pursue this material success as part of a balanced life, but we recognise and acknowledge that this is only a small part of our success. If you are like me, you might be questioning many of the things you have done right up to this point in life.

This is a *good* thing. It means that you are waking up and becoming self-aware. You are now strengthening the belief that you will successfully redesign your mind. You are cultivating the belief that it is up to you to decide how you feel. Redefining your definition of success can make you more ambitious than ever. You might only need to slightly adjust your course, or you might need to change ships. Either way you can acknowledge that something in your life will change and that you hold the power to make it happen.

If you had the power to control your fate and select one of the three options below for your life, which one would you choose?

A) To be successful
B) To be rich
C) To be happy

I know my answer and it is amazingly simple isn't it? Answer C – to be happy is the only answer that really matters. You could be the most successful, or the richest person in the world – yet if you are not happy it doesn't mean shit. You could have nothing to your name and be the happiest person on the planet. Answer C is the only option that you can change with nothing other than your mind.

MOVE THE GOAL POSTS

Imagine what it would be like if you were playing a game where every time you reached the goal, the goal posts would automatically shift further away, keeping you chasing and chasing, without ever reaching the goal. It would be pretty frustrating wouldn't it? Are you doing this in your own life? I know I was. Whenever I would achieve something special, I would spend little time celebrating the success before I would say something like, 'Yeah, it was good but now I need to do X'. Or I would put myself down by saying that it was easy and anyone else could do it; or that this achievement was just a formality and nothing really special. No this was not a formality and what you achieved was special. You've just moved the goal posts. Of course you are not going to feel fulfilled if you don't acknowledge your achievements. Of course you are going to miss out on the joy and happiness if you do not soak up the positive aspect of what just happened. Of course you aren't going to be grateful because it feels like you never have anything to be grateful for. Life can be a challenge when the goal posts keep moving.

When we reach a goal we need to allow ourselves time to celebrate the goal. Give yourself a pat on the back and acknowledge the achievement. We need to celebrate the good times and accentuate the positive. Not enjoying the positives is a way of putting yourself down. You might have gone out on a good date and your mind is racing ahead thinking about whether she will want a second date, or if you will have sex, or if you will end up in a relationship (*slow down, Stef, they only just met*). You had a good date? Great! Enjoy the thought that you had an awesome date and that's it. The rest can wait. You just scored a goal by having an awesome date. Feel happy about what you just achieved and enjoy the moment. Leave the goal posts where they are, celebrate, and then put out a new set of goal posts after you have enjoyed the first taste of success.

MORE SEX PLEASE

Success is just like sex. *It doesn't happen often but when it does, those 2 minutes are the time of your life.* Jokes aside, what I was trying to say is that sex is just like success, or maybe success is just like sex? Either way the point is that you could have the best, spine tingling, erotic, wall-banging, climactic sex you have ever had (*now you're talking*); but no matter how good the sex was, not long after you are wanting to do it again. But why? You just had the *best sex ever*. Surely you don't need to ever do it again? Of course we do! No one says, 'Oh, that sex was so good that I'm never going to need to have sex again'. The fact is that even after this award-winning sex, if you go a certain period of time without it, you'll be begging for any type of sex.

Ok, now that we've all had a moment to cool off, the point is that no matter how good the sex (or success) is, we are never content and we always want more. Yes, as we get older our urges for sex and success may reduce, because we've had a lot of it by then (*you're kidding yourself Stef!*) Either way it is something that we need to understand that we will probably never stop wanting. This is why billionaires get up every morning and work a 15-hour day. Assuming you are not already a billionaire, if I gave you one billion dollars, do you think that you would work another day in your life? I highly doubt it. So why is it that once we hit one billion dollars we still keep working and still keep pushing for *more?* The reason is because there is no ceiling with success, money, or even sex. This is why most people never reach a point where they say that they are successful enough and stop chasing new goals. However, as discussed earlier we can redefine what success means to us.

For many ex-sports stars who are now retired and past their physical prime, those who cannot redefine what success means often end up depressed because they were unable to deal with the progression of their life. Their environment changed (due to retirement, injury or being delisted). The only way they failed was to not change their mindset and move forward with their life. They were stuck in the 'living in the past' cognitive distortion – more on cognitive distortions later. Those who are able to transfer their success into other areas like coaching, commentating, working for charity or finding a new passion are much more likely to live the rest of their lives with happiness and potentially more success – whatever that means to them.

GUILTY AS CHARGED

Are you feeling guilty that you put yourself first? This is another challenge of mine that I've faced time and time again; particularly because I am part of an Australian-Italian family and group of friends who always put family and friends first. Living as part of a group of people who will always put others first can put thoughts of guilt in your own mind if you want to put yourself first at times. I know it sounds silly but sometimes you might have to stay home and study instead of going to visit everyone who wants to see you. And sometimes you might just want to stay at home and watch a movie instead of going to an event that means so much to someone else. I still have feelings of guilt; however they have reduced dramatically since I redesigned my mind. We can only be at one place at a time, doing one thing at a time. Whilst it would be awesome to be in two places at once, we need to accept the reality that if we are working towards a goal, it means that we are going to miss out on things from time to time. There is always a cost. This doesn't mean that you are a bad person; it just means that you have other things in your life that are more of a priority at that time. Just like the graph I showed you in a previous chapter, we have to keep the balance to maintain our happiness. Everyone's balance will be different and we need to understand this. Someone might allocate more time to family where you might allocate at lot less time to this area of your life. That's totally cool, but this doesn't mean that we need to feel guilty because we choose not to dedicate as much time or energy to our family life.

Here's another language redesign that you may want to consider. I have chosen to remove the word 'can't' and replace it with 'won't'. It's amazing how changing just one word can make a massive difference. How often does someone ask us to do something but we have too much to do and we say, 'I can't go'. This makes you feel guilty and powerless. You feel as though you want to go but you *can't*. It leaves you feeling that the decision is out of your control. By changing this to 'won't' it gives you the power back. You feel empowered that you made the decision. It doesn't mean that you respond like a dick, but it means that you are in control of your life. You can add to the sentence to help give the person another option to ensure that they still feel valued. For example you can comfortably say, 'I won't be able to make it today, how about next Thursday?' This brings some of the control back into your life and removes the sense of you being flapped around in the wind at the control of someone else. Remember that if you want to spend your Saturday on the couch in your underwear watching Netflix while a group of your friends are going to a social event, this is totally fine because it is *your* life. There is no need to feel guilty or as if you are self-indulging, because the people going to the social event are self-indulging too; they feel good by going to the event – and if they don't feel good about going and still attend to avoid feelings of guilt, well aren't they the silly ones then?

CHAPTER EIGHT
THE RIGHT ENVIRONMENT

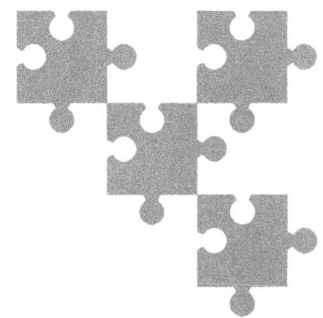

Sometimes we do all the right things and have all the right behaviours, but things still don't work out. Sometimes we need to change our environment. The Buddha talks about The Noble Eightfold Path which has influenced me during the redesign of my mind. You may want to research these teachings and see if they apply to you. The best thing about Buddhism is that the Buddha's teachings and learnings are so practical, making it easy to apply to our generation. I am not a Buddhist but I love many of the practices and teachings. The Buddha explains the *Right Livelihood* which is probably the closest thing that I can compare to having the right environment. Right Livelihood talks about having the right job and way to earn a living. Building on this we can add where you live, where you work, and who your friends are as factors of the right environment.

MONEY DOESN'T GROW ON TREES

In my home city of Adelaide there is a shopping centre that decided to enclose a magnificent tree inside the centre. They spent millions on making a glass ceiling for the tree so that it had sun to help it grow. They spent so much time and money on this tree. The tree had all of the nutrients, water and sun it could ever wish for, and yet after a short period of time, the tree died. One alleged reason for the death of the tree was that there wasn't sufficient oxygen levels inside for the tree to live. For a small city of Adelaide this was a massive news story and an embarrassment for the shopping centre. Whilst it was a sad story for the tree (*and also the person who brought up the idea of enclosing a magnificent tree*), one thing we can learn from this is that no matter how much time, effort, thinking, planning and most importantly money goes into something, it doesn't mean that it will continue to live. Even a magnificent tree that had many of the things it needs to live can in fact die if it is in the *wrong environment*. We also need to live in the *Right Environment*.

The right environment is so important to our overall happiness and as we learnt from the tree, no matter how good our mindset is, if we are in the wrong environment, then we are certainly heading for death. It also taught me that hindsight is a beautiful thing. I am sure there was much planning and research put into the success of the tree - but they got it wrong. Looking back now I am sure everyone thinks it was a silly idea, but aren't many of our decisions considered silly in hindsight?

The story of the tree can be related to my own life. When I was anxious and depressed after my holiday in the US – I put this down to me not having the *Right Mindset*. Without making any change, after some time I eventually fell into the *Right Mindset*. This foolishly and incorrectly led to me believing that I was in the w*rong environment* and that the answer was to change my environment. My job was no longer fulfilling, travel would only make me sick and disappoint me, and I concluded that changing my environment and taking a big risk with a new business was the right answer. Just like the story of the tree, looking back now this seemed like a silly decision that I *should* have seen coming. Hindsight is a beautiful thing. Not long into my own business I found out that it wasn't my environment that needed to change; all along it was my mindset that needed to change. Now that I had my own business it was actually *my environment* that further contributed to the feelings of anxiety and depression. Just like the tree in the shopping centre, I had most of the right intentions but by being in the wrong environment this caused me to suffer. In the end I realised that I had a great deal of work to do as I had to change both my environment and my mindset. The funny thing is that there are times that I work harder than I did when I had the business, yet now with both the right mindset and the right environment, life is much better.

I hope this story of the poor shopping centre tree empowers you to think that it's never too late to change your environment. If you are reading this book it means that you must be alive, and therefore you have time to redesign your life. I know that making a change of environment will be much easier for some. For me, even though it was physically easy to make the change to close my business and move on to something else – mentally it was a massive challenge. I know that change is not easy. Others may find it physically hard. If you have a husband and two kids you might find it a challenge to retire as a mother and move out to Las Vegas as a party promoter. *Notice how I didn't say can't or won't?* This is because I didn't want to remove the empowerment of the decision from you because only you can decide what you want to do with your life and what is right and wrong for *you*. Maybe you can change your environment another way that still involves your family? This is something only you can work out as you work on the redesign of your mind.

YOU'RE ONLY AS GOOD AS THE COMPANY YOU KEEP

Even though I have had most of the same friends for most of my life; I have chosen to spend more of my time with the ones that are in my *right environment*. Maybe you have some friends or family that are not providing you with what you need. These are some challenging questions you need to ask yourself. Yes, the comfort of a life-long friend is something important to everyone, but if they are bringing out negative energy or not helping you on your journey to happiness, then is it really worth it?

Again, you need to ask yourself *does it really matter?* Your friends and family must compliment who you are as a person, and if they don't then I would say it may be a good time to consider how much time you want to spend with them. For example, if you are trying to cut back on drinking alcohol and all of your friends go out and get drunk every weekend, well then maybe you might not want to spend as much time with them. Or maybe you could change *when* you see your friends. Instead of meeting up on a Saturday night (when everyone is ready to get drunk), you could meet them for lunch. Small changes like this can help you maintain your friendships without having to be in an environment that is not right for you.

CULTIVATE YOUR GARDEN…OR FIND A NEW ONE

Is your work totally fulfilling, or at least leading you on a path that will get you to the fulfilling work you want to do? I say this because sometimes we need to endure the *wrong* environment as a pathway to get to the *right* environment. We cannot expect that we can just move into the top position at work without having to earn our position. Maybe this wrong environment is actually the right environment (because it leads to the right environment), and you just need to show some grit and stick it out. Just like the tree, if you are not in the job that is right for you, or at least leading you to the right path, then you may want to think about changing jobs. I was one of those people that endured the wrong environment for no reason, turning up to work every day, putting up with the challenges that I was facing for a goal that was not in line with who I truly was.

I often hear others complaining about their jobs, what is wrong with their boss, or the amount of work they have to do, or that they have no career options. Well if there is something wrong with your job, then why not *change* it? I know it is a challenge but it may be the best thing you ever do. If you say that you 'can't' change, maybe you need to ask yourself if this is due to your mindset. Are you really saying that you *won't* change? Is it because deep down you know that you like the money that you are making (even if it means you have to be unhappy)? These are the questions that you need to ask yourself to find out if there is a genuine reason why you 'won't change' jobs, or if it's just a bullshit excuse that you tell yourself to make sense of why you are turning up every day to a job that sucks. I know that finding the right environment is not an easy task. I didn't just wake up one day and say, 'Oh *yes, I am ready to close my business and apply for a new job'*. Redesigning your life takes time and change takes commitment. Commitment to investigating what it is that you actually want from life.

Changing environment requires a lot of thought and understanding of your values and beliefs. You need to figure out what the most important things in your life are and then work out if your job is the right environment for this life. Remember that changing environment and changing mindset are the two major things we can focus on changing in our lives; everything else is pretty much out of our control and we need to accept what happens. Accepting that our environment is shit and doing nothing about it is a choice that we might have to live with. No matter how good your mindset is, you owe it to yourself to set up the right environment to get the most out of your new mindset. The difference between you and that poor shopping centre tree is that the tree didn't have a choice. The tree is planted in its roots and cannot make the choice on whether it wants to stay or pack up its shit and move to Mexico. But we do have this choice. Yes, we have metaphorical roots in our environments, but know that if it is physically possible, then you can do it. You are in control of where you live your life. As I have explained throughout the book, nothing is stopping you from being who you want to be other than your own mind. If the tree could talk to you, what would it say to you about your problems with your environment? Would the tree say that we are acting ridiculously because it is physically so easy for us to pack up and change environments whilst the tree is stuck without choice? It is time to stop limiting yourself and start setting your own limitations as to what is possible and what is not.

GOD, HELP ME

There are a lot of people who believe in a God and living by a set of values that may take you to heaven in the afterlife. Unfortunately this book has no answers as to whether this is true or not but one thing I do believe is that praying to God will not change the future events of your life. I am a Catholic and I would like to think that there is a God up there somewhere – but I'm not sure. If praying to God was the way to find happiness then we could all be easily saved. I say that we need to work on cultivating our own happiness. Yes, you can have faith; however, from my experience I don't believe that praying to God, asking for something to change in your life is going to result in an empowered, positive mindset. I am not going to go into the history of religion and discuss the possibility of God's power, but I believe that it is up to us to make good things happen. Pray to God for faith and inner strength if you are religious; however everything else is up to you to make happen.

Religious leaders and society have influenced us to believe that praying to God during tough times will help us. It wasn't long ago when we would make sacrifices to God in the hope of receiving rain for our farmers, or a prosperous time ahead, yet science has come a long way since then and fully debugged this myth. We need to understand that whilst we can pray to God as a matter of faith, we cannot rely on God to make things better. If God is up there pulling the strings of our fate, would God give you the result you want just by asking for it in a prayer? Or would God want you to work for it? This is one of the fundamental reasons why I believe that no matter what your faith is, you are in control of how your mind works and how you cultivate your emotions. By praying to God and asking for happiness, or to be free of depression or anxiety, you are removing the power from yourself. By accepting and acknowledging that our negative emotions are a result of our own mind, we can then empower ourselves to take action and work on changing our mind. You need to put in the hard work to cultivate a positive mindset and find the right environment. If there is a heaven, I would assume that being a good person would help you gain entry when the time comes. The first thing you can do to be a good person is to be good to yourself. So let's leave fate of the universe up to God or whoever else is in charge and work on what we can control by cultivating the right mindset by moving forward on our journey to redesign our mind.

Dear God, if you are reading this I apologise for everything. I am just trying to empower people to live a happier life on their own account and I will pay for my sins when I meet you at the golden gates. Hopefully not for a while yet! P.S. Mum wants me to find a girlfriend, do you know anyone? Much love, Stef.

EMBRACING MEDITATION

Meditation will change your life. There is no doubt about it. Meditation is a powerful tool that you can use to help you calm your mind when things are moving too fast. I think I have one of the fasted minds around. My mind is great for quickly adding up figures in my head, being witty at parties and thinking quickly on the job. What my mind is not great at doing is trying to relax when I am anxious or worked up about something. Meditation has helped me slow down my mind to a manageable pace. I know that meditation can be scary, especially if you have a fast mind like mine. But the reality is that we are the people who get the most out of it! I think of the mind as being like a spinning wheel, and for those who have a fast mind, well it is not healthy to have that thing spinning at 10,000 RPM all the time.

One part of the redesign of our mind is rewriting our thought processes so that we have the right thoughts (or right responses to negative thoughts) coming into our mind. We are working on this by rewriting our thoughts. The second part is allowing our mind to relax and slow down every once in a while. Kind of like putting your computer on sleep mode when you don't need it. There are thousands of meditations available online which can help you in every situation. Go to my website wellnessofhealth.com for information on the latest meditation apps that can help you on your journey. . Practicing a mind calming meditation twice a day will change your life. By finding just 15 minutes in the morning and 15 minutes in the evening you will make a massive difference to the clarity of your mind, assisting you to better focus and cope with the challenges of life.

USING MEDITATION TO CALM THE MIND

A simple meditation you can practice to help slow down and calm your mind is a breathing meditation. Let's try it now. Find a quiet spot in the house or at work and get rid of all your distractions. Your phone and television will be the most important things to switch off. You want to have at least 15 minutes for this meditation to truly feel the power of meditation. Set a timer if you like. Sit in an upright, comfortable position and close your eyes. With your eyes closed, focus on your breathing. Feel the air come in through your nostrils, into your lungs and then back out again. Watch as it goes in and out. See what you can pay attention to and anything that you notice. Maybe you feel your bottom sitting on your chair, your feet on the floor or the clothes on your skin. Sit and continue to watch your breath as much as possible. Watch it go in and out. Allow your body to take care of you while you rest your mind. You are not going to sleep; you are totally aware and awake, watching your breathing.

Now it won't take long for thoughts to rush in. Probably a few seconds if you are anything like me! This is totally normal and ok. The trick, which takes much practice to master, is to watch the thoughts and not entertain them. You will find at first that a thought will come in and you will continue to engage with it. *What am I going to cook for dinner tonight? Maybe chicken. I had chicken last night so I need to do something else. I wonder if I have any spinach in the fridge. That will go well with chicken. Oh wait, I am not cooking chicken tonight silly me. Wait, I am meant to be meditating. Shit!* This can go on for a long time if you don't catch yourself. Laugh about it and start again. Aim to watch your thoughts as if they are passing by on a river. You are the observer of your breath, and any thoughts that come in will just go sailing by. You have time after meditation to engage your thoughts but for now your job is to watch your breath and rest your mind.

Do not get angry or disappointed with yourself as the thoughts run in. Allow them to be. Practice, practice, practice. 15 minutes will actually feel like a long time. The most important part of meditation is not to give up. Do it again and again. Your meditation is helping you de-clutter and relax your mind, even if it feels like it got worse when you first started. This is just the wheel of your mind slowing down and freaking out because it isn't being engaged like it has been for many years. Practice this morning and night if you can, and anytime that you are feeling particularly anxious or overwhelmed. I find that even a quick 5-minute meditation at lunch or when things get really busy, can make a massive difference. You owe it to yourself to find time to relax your mind. Once you are ready you may like to practice a more spiritual meditation to help you find out more about who you are.

USING MEDITATION TO FIND YOUR HIGHER SELF

There is lots of research available on the different parts of our brain and the workings of the mind. Some believe in the 1st brain and the 2nd brain; some talk about the conscious and the subconscious; some talk about our mind and our soul; some talk about our self and our higher self; and finally, Austin Powers talks about him and his 'mojo'. Whilst I think everyone has (and can lose) their mojo, one major change for me was to get in touch with my higher self. I wasn't always a spiritual person but I found that finding my higher self has helped me on my journey of becoming a person and better aligning my life to where I want it to be. I know it will help you too if you can allow yourself to read with an open mind throughout the next section.

Everyone will have their own perception of their own higher-self. What I believe is that your higher self is your higher consciousness, something you can speak to, hear, and listen to. In meditation I often like to seek advice from my higher self. In our day to day lives we are often on autopilot, just doing what needs to be done without any reference to our higher self, or why we are actually doing what we are doing. Some people *wake up* ten years later and realise that they have been on autopilot the whole time. We need to find our higher self because our higher self has the answers of where and what we *truly* want to be. Our higher self is like someone who is always there for you, guiding you along the way. It might be like a mentor, a friend, you in the future, you as an older person, you as a different being, an ancient monk, anything. You will know when you meet your higher self. My dealings with my higher self feel like talking to someone that is you, and also knows everything about you. Your higher self can tell you whether you are on the right path or not. Your higher self can make you accountable for your recent actions. Are you behaving the way you want to behave? Are your actions helping you achieve your goals, or are they hindering you? Our higher self can help us cut the crap because deep down, past the autopilot, past all the bullshit, we often already know the answers to the questions we have. Our higher self will help us clear our mind and find those answers. We can use a form of meditation to help find our higher self. For those that haven't practiced mediation before, or have tried and failed – that is ok. It is time for us to open our minds and try something new, or try something that we have failed at in the past and give it another go.

CHAPTER EIGHT – THE RIGHT ENVIRONMENT

When you are ready, let's meditate and find your higher self. Find a quiet spot in the house or at work and remove all your distractions. You probably need about 15 minutes to do this meditation so make sure that you have the time. Put on some headphones and set up some peaceful mediation music that has no words or singing. Next you need to sit and get yourself into a comfortable position. Close your eyes and allow yourself to ease into a meditation. Relax and allow your thoughts to flow in and out. Even the most experienced will have thoughts running through their head, just let them pass. Do not force them out, just watch them go by. Now for the next few minutes, focus on your breath. Breathe in for three counts and then breathe out for four counts. This will slow and calm your breathing pattern. After a few minutes, you can stop controlling and start watching your breathing. Feel your body breathe in and out as time goes on without you thinking about it. *How amazing is it that your body knows to breathe in and out without you having to do anything?* Your body is caring for you and looking after your health. Keep watching your breath and letting your thoughts float by. A negative thought may come in, *it's ok*. Just watch it and let it pass. You can rewrite your negative thoughts afterwards if you need to.

After about five minutes you are now ready to find your higher self. I'm sure that you are full of anticipation, wonder and maybe even uncertainty. That's ok and it is all part of the process. You may need to read the next part a few times before you practice it in your own mind. Picture yourself trekking up a mountain. You might have people with you or you might be alone. It's not an easy trek but you know you are trekking to meet your higher self. You need to speak with your higher self and this is the only way to get there. The path might be a challenging one, or it might be easier. When you do this again later, things that you associate in your life will affect your path. You might find that you do not know where you're going, or it is taking you longer, or that you are sore, or hurt, or tired etc; these will all be things you can relate back to what is going on in your life.

We continue down the path. You know why you are trekking but you have no idea what your higher self will look like and what your higher self will have to say. Finally you reach a set of doors at the top of this trek. What the doors lead to is up to you; it could be a house, a castle, a monastery, a church, a hall, a hut, a shelter, anything. Now you open these large doors and walk inside. You continue to walk until you find your higher self sitting down, exactly as you are right now, looking back at you, smiling, as if he, she or it has been waiting for you this whole time. Your higher self knew that you were coming even though you never said anything. Your higher self is already enlightened, wise and knows everything about you, because your higher self is a part of you. Kind of like looking at a future self with all of the life experiences you have now, plus another 50 years. You are seeking the advice of your higher self. You now have only a few minutes with your higher self and you can ask your higher self a few questions. There may be something that is on your mind from your own life. You instantly know what questions you want to ask your higher self. You ask them and they smile and give you the answer. If you are not happy with something in your life maybe your higher self will show disappointment or frustration. Or maybe your higher self will be kind and caring and supportive. You want to ask your higher self even more but you don't have much time before you have to go away; and you'll have to wait until next time. After a short time you will say goodbye to your higher self and thank it, coming back to your sitting position, to where you are now, watching your breath, feeling the presence of the room, the walls around you and where you are right now. Well done, you have just met your higher self!

If the above didn't work for you it is up to you to work out what you need to change. Were there any distractions? Were you not in the right mindset? Was your mind busy or closed? Did you give yourself enough time to settle? You might not know the answer as to why it didn't work but this is ok because you can try again. For the rest of you I am sure that you got a taste of what it is like to speak with your higher self and get guidance from yourself. This is a meditation that can truly help shed some light on how we feel about where we are in life and where we want to go. Maybe thoughts will come up of items that you haven't yet addressed from your past. It may be time to work on these things by rewriting your thoughts, talking with someone you trust or even seeing a psychologist (personal trainer for your mind). This meditation can really help you change your life. In my own dealings with my higher self, sometimes my higher self is not happy with me because I have the wrong mindset. At other times my higher self is kind to me and helps me through a challenging time.

Your relationship with your higher self is for you and only you. Nothing you say or do with your higher self is right or wrong; it is for you to help yourself on your journey and find out things about your own life that may be covered up by the day to day bullshit we have to deal with. Maybe it's been hard to figure out what we truly wanted in the past because we are so tunnel-visioned by the rat race that we do not take time to sit back and reflect. Now is the time to reflect and this short meditation can really help you, just as it has helped me. Remember that you need to be open-minded because it's not possible for a meditation of this nature to work if your mind *won't* allow it. You are now well and truly on the way to redesigning your mind. You are now spending time in the mind-gym, lifting heavier and heavier weights for your mind. You are sparking transformation and helping yourself cultivate a life that you want to live. Remember that *the man who moves mountains starts by moving the smallest stone*. Without even knowing it, you have already moved many stones on your own journey to move mountains. Well done, keep going!

CHAPTER NINE
WHAT CAN I DO TO CHANGE

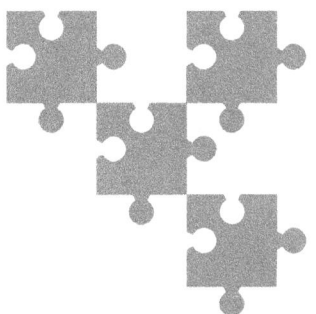

The thing about redesigning your mind is that you have to *want* to change. Once you have decided that you want to change and believe that it is possible, your mind will listen to you and redesigning will be possible. Are you willing to do what it takes to get yourself in the best mental state possible or do you just want it to happen? Redesigning your mind involves taking yourself out of your comfort zone and doing things that you never thought you would have done. Ultimately the decision is yours as to how far you take it – but I made a promise to myself to keep searching to find a way to continuously cultivate my own happiness.

IS IT JUST A PLACEBO?

I have done a lot of research into the placebo effect. I have no doubt that the placebo effect has some role to play in how successful the redesign of your mind will be. Whether something is a placebo or not, ask yourself the question – does it really matter if something only works as a placebo? If you feel like something is working then does it matter if it is *actually* working, or just the thought of what you are doing that makes you feel better? I say who cares! Just like the bottle of 'Michael's Secret Stuff' in the movie *Space Jam;* it is amazing what challenges we and the Looney Tunes Squad can overcome just by 'thinking' that something will work. Learn to have an open mind to things and let down your walls of scepticism before you even try it for yourself. If eating chocolate is 'clinically proven' not to increase happiness, then why would anyone eat it? Because people *think* chocolate makes them happy. Chocolate *tastes* good and it *feels* good when you are eating it. If it makes you happy, then it works. Everything in the world has a different effect on every person, so why not find out for yourself if a certain change is for you? Whether it is a placebo or not, the resulting *emotion* will be the same – so you might as well embrace it and let someone else decide whether it is a placebo or not.

PRACTICING YOGA

When I first started yoga I thought it was only for green-smoothie-drinking women in active wear – but thankfully I was wrong. On the first day I went to yoga class I felt like a little boy going to his first day of school. Here I was going into class with a bunch of well, fit females, flexible, confident, able and ready to put me to shame on the yoga mat. *Talk about getting out of your comfort zone.* My confidence was also at an all-time low; I had lost a lot of weight, had no energy, and looked (and was) physically and mentally drained. However I had an urge to try something that may help me and yoga was next on the list. I thought the girls might be thinking, 'What is wrong with this guy and why is he even here?' The great thing about this was I learnt more about myself and my insecurities. It was true that I cared more about what everyone around me thought about me. This was a thought that I could later write out and redesign.

I quickly learned that yoga is about challenging yourself and having your own experience on the mat; not about comparing yourself to others. By practicing yoga you will learn that everything you experience on the mat is totally relatable to where you are in life. My first few weeks brought it all out and I was physically and mentally exhausted by the end of each session. I felt as if I had given everything I had to give and that I wasn't getting anywhere. I would often give up during the poses – with the excuse that I was 'not experienced enough'. I realised that this was how I was behaving in life. When things were challenging, I would 'drop the pose', and make an excuse.

Yoga has helped me challenge my own mind and develop mental and physical strength. At first I would often lose my balance, putting it down to my 'dizziness' and other psychosomatic symptoms I had made up in my mind. One day after class I was chatting with one of my teachers about 'how hard it was' as a male to practice yoga – and she kindly told me that I was being silly and that it was 'all in my head'. My balance was off because my mind was not balanced. My strength was low because my mind saw me as a weak person. This was another bit of learning that I had to accept. *Who knew a yoga teacher could be so wise!* Eventually I got stronger in both the mind and body, and yoga became fun. Yoga has taught me to live in the moment. When you are practicing yoga on the mat, this is where you are. If your mind is elsewhere, you will fall over, just like in real life.

Yogis will agree that the biggest challenge with yoga is turning up to the mat. I now think this has a lot to do with many of the other things in life.

Turning up is half of the battle. Having a positive mindset when you get there is the other half. Yes, yoga will take you out of your comfort zone – but that is exactly the point. It will bring you out into the public arena, challenging you to face your fears and grow.

PRACTICING MINDFULNESS

Mindfulness is about throwing yourself into the present moment without any thoughts of the past or future. Mindfulness is a form of meditation that when practiced will help slow your spinning mind. Mindfulness is one of my biggest challenges still today as I am always ready to think about the 100 things I want to do. *Ok, I need to keep writing my book, tonight I have a birthday party to go to, I have to reply to that girl on Tinder, shit I forgot that I have to go shopping this morning, how good was that movie last night, hmm what will I cook for dinner, oh shit what about the book I need to keep writing.* Does this sound familiar? I was the worst at keeping my mind constantly spinning; and what makes it worse is that when those with a fast mind go through times of depression or anxiety, these running thoughts are usually negative ones, and hence why we spiral even more.

When I was in my greatest state of being overwhelmed, the thoughts were coming thick and fast and I couldn't escape them. Like I talked about earlier, doing the dishes nearly resulted in me blowing a fuse. It's hard to focus, your mind is foggy, you can't think straight and you can't enjoy yourself. Mindfulness will help in your quest for slowing down your mind – which goes hand in hand with everything else that we have talked about. Not only will we have better thought processes, but the frequency and constant drive of thought will slow down.

Let's practice being mindful now. Assuming that you're sitting down, feel yourself sitting in the chair, feel the weight of your body on the seat or couch. Feel your feet on the floor, feel your feet touching the surface of your thong (*Australian for flip-flop. Please get your mind out of the gutter you Americans*), feel your sock or shoe, feel the skin of your foot touching the surface. Feel your hands touching the book, feel your breath going in and out. Feel the tenseness in your shoulders; see if you can let them fall down and relax. Now rub your hand up and down your arm slowly, listen to the sound that it makes, and truly listen. Feel your hand against your arm; you've never *felt* this before. Without any thought other than what you are doing. Now I want you to be aware of the foot, your body, your bum on the couch, your breathing, your hand and the rubbing all at the same time. This is being truly mindful and present. You can apply this to everything that you do in life, including eating an apple. Try it!

The more you practice mindfulness the more in touch with the present you will be. For example, if you are anxious about walking into a room full of people that you don't know, be mindful of your clothes sitting on your body, *listen* to the sounds coming from the room, feel your feet walking on the floor, listen to your breath. Buddhism talks about the quest for enlightenment and how mindfulness plays a part. Ironically one way to help with mindfulness and being present is to set aside some time for thinking about things. Writing them on a piece of paper is even better. Take some time to 'think' and if you have anything that pops into your head outside of this 'thinking time' then quickly jot it down on your phone or a piece of paper for later. For the rest of your time you can be present and mindful of whatever task it is that you are doing. Take it to the next level and be mindful of when you are not being mindful. This self-awareness will help you free yourself from paying attention to the constant chatter in your mind.

REDESIGNING YOUR ENERGY

I cannot stress enough the power of positive energy. If your energy is negative, you are going to attract negative people, circumstances and emotions. If your energy is positive, you are going to attract the opposite. Yes, the law of attraction is something that has been much publicised, but do you actually live and breathe it? I know that I wasn't. Changing the frequency of my energy from negative to positive has had a tremendous effect on both my life and my happiness. If you wake up in the morning and start with a negative mindset about the day that lies ahead of you, then your day is going to feel like a slow burn that comes to a depressing end. If your energy is positively charged, looking for opportunities to create the day that you want to have, then positive things are going to happen. Try it. Sure, shit happens but it is how you react to the shit that is going to affect what you do next. Writing out your thoughts is going to help you move to a positive frequency, but you have to believe and have a desire to be positive. Set your tone to positive and never look back. Negative is not for you anymore. Win, lose or draw you are going to be positive and optimistic about what lies ahead in the future that you will create.

Now that you have set the tone of your energy to positive, it is time to *find your energy*. I remember years ago I use to say that I didn't want to walk anywhere. I didn't like to expend much energy and always took the easy way. In hindsight this tells me a lot about who I used to be. I used to always say that 'I have no energy' and I couldn't imagine how anyone would find the energy to do all this exercise that we *should* do in a day. Are you depressed and saying that you don't have the energy to do anything? I know what it's like. Usually whenever I get a bill, letter, or email, I always action it that day or the next day at the latest, paying any bills and taking any action required. Yes, there's a little OCD in me, but I don't feel the need to change it, so I *won't*. However, when I was depressed I couldn't 'find the energy' to pay a bill or open any of my letters. I remember receiving a late payment notice for a bill. I was ashamed that I had let this happen (further fuelling the depressive causing thoughts). *How could I climb this mountain with no energy, how could I pay all these bills, I am a loser.* I was putting off taking any action as I was waiting for my energy levels to come back. After I drew the line in the sand and got off the couch and picked up one letter and paid one late bill, I knew that I had found my energy. I was now creating my own energy and responsible for my actions. I was no longer a victim of low energy. It wasn't long before things started to change for the better. Paying this one late bill had inspired me to move mountains. As Confucius said, 'The man who moves mountains starts by moving just one stone'.

I know it's a challenge, and I'm sure you may be sighing all the time if you are depressed, just like I was. You may be struggling and not wanting to rollover and get up, or get out of your pyjamas, but I can tell you that getting out of bed and getting changed is the first step to charging your energy levels. Yes, you can do it; I know you can. I was in the absolutely lowest state of energy where getting out of bed felt like climbing a mountain but eventually you have to decide to take action. Do something right now, anything to boost your energy. Get changed, clean the kitchen bench, go for a walk, call a friend, anything. This will kick-start the motor that creates your energy. This will also help fuel your positive thoughts and help pull you out of your depression. No longer are you a victim of depression, you are now someone taking action and moving forward with your life. Even if you aren't depressed, you can still find another gear of energy that you thought never existed by inspiring more positivity and action towards your goals.

When I beat my depression and was living by my redesigned mind, my energy levels went through the roof. I went from helplessly lying on the couch to working full time, while completing a master's degree, living on my own again and staying in touch with friends. I also managed to fit in a trip to Europe as well. I finished a 12 week master's course in three weeks (with top marks) to make this Europe trip happen. When I was in Europe I would walk all over a city all day and party all night. Flash back to when I was depressed and lying on the couch and I wouldn't have thought a life like this was even possible! I had successfully redesigned my mind and was now full of the energy that I once lacked. Sure, an experience like going to Europe is going to boost your energy levels, but this is exactly my point. You don't receive an injection with a shot of energy at customs when you land in Europe. Your mind creates the energy as you are excited and entertained by the life-changing experiences that you are about to have.

Recently I had a friend who experienced depression. This friend had no understanding of how hard depression had been when I went through it. This friend told me years before his depression that I just had to 'snap out of it and stop worrying'. If only depression was that simple. This friend was once one of the most active people I know. He had a passion for life and was very proud of his independence. What happened next was that his life took a turn for the worse and he was dependent on others for a period of time. Depression came next. It wasn't due to the lack of support or assistance while being dependent – but due to his negative mindset about the situation. As he spiralled downward I saw a lot of myself when I went through my depression. He lost all of his energy in an instant. My friend told me one day that he finally understood how I had felt when I was depressed. He now understood how debilitating depression could be. Eventually my friend got better. I cannot claim much of the credit because as we know, depression is a battle that you have to fight. We can have all the guidance and support in the world but it is up to us to turn the page. My friend now has a different outlook and can appreciate how depression can leave you feeling powerless and weak. Whether you are depressed or just low on energy, I urge you to take action and find your energy because an active, optimistic, positively attuned person will not stay depressed for long.

Trust me when I say that every little thing you do will help build your energy. Call that friend, go out for coffee, pay that bill, brush your teeth, have a shower, get your hair or nails done (boys included), go see that funny movie that might make you laugh, text that other guy or girl, cook your own dinner. Take action now. You will have to get moving too. Exercise is unbelievably good at changing how you feel both physically and mentally. Do you feel weak, low on energy or powerless? Time to get active and build your energy. Watch your energy levels rise and your psychosomatic symptoms disappear when you get moving! Do anything to get your body moving and blood pumping. Set your tone to positive energy, then go out and do something that makes you sweat and get your energy levels charged. Take action on what it is that you want to do in life. Empower yourself to be responsible for your own life and watch how you will now be ready to take on any challenge.

COUNT THE LITTLE WINS

Do you only care about the big goals? Finishing that university degree; getting married; getting that promotion? Yes these are all great things but in reality these magical events don't happen very often. All of these events involve living in the future. Previously I only cared about the big wins and everything else was irrelevant. No wonder I ended up *depressed*. Now I implement a thought called 'counting the little wins'. It doesn't matter how small the win is, but you can count a win as a win. It's a great way to pump yourself up. When I was down and out, opening that first letter was a little win. *Great work Stef, you've opened one letter!* When I got my new job after my business closed I celebrated the fact that I got a job; previously I would have been anxious about whether I would be good at the job or not, or if I would keep my job, or if the other staff would like me. Someone out there thought, *You know what; I like this Stef bloke and what he has to offer, let's give him a job.* How good is that! Count the small wins. *You made it to lunch? Great work! A whole first day without blowing anything up? Awesome*! Go home and celebrate. Who gives a shit if you didn't win a noble prize; you can still be happy about yourself and your one day of achievements. Why not feel good about it instead of disqualifying the positive? Did you sign up to a gym? Celebrate! Enjoy the journey and remember that *the man who moves mountains starts by moving just one stone.* Start counting the little wins and watch the positive emotions flow. Say to yourself 'that's a little win' whenever it happens. Your mind loves hearing that you are 'winning' and having 'wins', regardless of the size.

REDESIGNING YOUR DIET

Oh no, not a diet! I know, I know. Going on a diet kind of sucks, but maybe that's because you've told yourself that. Maybe going on a diet could be exciting, empowering, fulfilling, and maybe even fun. Hopefully this is another example of how different thoughts will lead to different emotions.

I have tried numerous diets over the years. Protein shakes, meal replacements, fasting, intermittent fasting, low carb, high carb, high fat, low fat, vegan, vegetarian, carnivore (no humans), caveman, and even paleo have all been trialled. Whilst I am no dietician, the results are pretty clear to me and my main result is that a *balanced* diet is the key to a healthy diet; but what is a balanced diet? And what is balanced for me will probably be totally out of balance for you; so I do believe that going to see a doctor or dietician and getting a meal plan written up will be a great way to help you on the journey to redesign your life.

In my unprofessional opinion I believe that a balanced diet basically means as little 'processed' foods as possible and as many vegetables as possible. This *should* not come as a shock to you. Do you really think that we were made to eat processed foods and high amounts of sugar and processed meats? You can imagine what it was like as an Italian boy when I told Mum and Nonna that I wanted to cut back on pizza, prosciutto and gelato! After they both woke up from what they thought was a bad dream, they shook their head in disappointment and we had a laugh about it. *Redesigning* our diet is part of the change in lifestyle that we need. Redesigning your diet doesn't mean that you have to give up the things you love; it might just mean that you change how often you have them. I will always enjoy a burger and a few drinks on the weekend. Yes, eating a block of chocolate feels good while you're doing it, but what does it do for your happiness in the long run? Energy drinks are also something to steer away from as often as possible because they can have a similar effect to an amphetamine. These drinks trigger a fast racing mind and cause your anxiety to rise. Remember that you can boost your own energy by doing the right things with your mind and exercise – and leave the energy drinks for those who need wings. You don't need me to tell you what foods are good and bad for you – I am sure that deep down you *know* what is good and bad, it's just a matter of finding the balance that is right for you. Be kind to your body, your gut and yourself. Remember that the mind-body connection is more powerful than you think and the foods that you ingest will ultimately play a part in how you feel about yourself.

Some of the most challenging times of depression and anxiety for me came after big weekends on the booze. Alcohol is like throwing fuel on your fire of negative thoughts and I would suggest that if you are in a low point to limit your alcohol consumption. Still have a drink or two but a weekend bender is a no, no. There is plenty of time to have a few too many drinks when you are feeling great again. One thing I struggled with is that I imposed an alcohol ban on myself which was too harsh at the time. A lot of our socialising is done around alcohol and I must say that cutting it out didn't work for me. At the time I went too far and locked myself away from many social events because of the fear of alcohol. When I did go out and someone asked me if I wanted a drink, I looked at them as if they had just asked me if I wanted a glass of poison – this made things worse for me at the time as I felt alienated and as if I didn't fit in anymore. Because I didn't allow myself to drink, this caused negative thoughts around enjoying myself with a few drinks and temporarily set me back. Remember to be kind to yourself and *maintain the balance*. Don't be scared of a few casual drinks out with friends.

BEND LIKE THE WILLOW TREE

The story of the oak and willow trees has massive relevance to the flexibility of our minds. An oak tree is strong, holds its ground and has little bend, while the willow tree sways whichever way the wind blows. If the winds of change are strong enough, the oak tree will snap and break as it has no give, while the willow tree will go on pleasantly and move back to its original position as soon as the wind dies down.

Are you stiff and strong like an oak tree or do you bend like a willow tree? In other words, how do you react when things do not go to plan? Nearly every day in your life something will not go to plan. Sure, we can let the small things slide, but how do you go about bending when the winds get strong enough to break you? I know that I grew up stiffer than an oak tree. When things were great, I was strong and tall. When things didn't go to plan, I would snap. Learning to be flexible is a massive way to reduce stress and increase your happiness. The willow tree does not stress that the wind is blowing to the East; the willow tree says, '*Yeah sure, I will bend that way today*'. The oak tree stands strong and suffers due to its inflexibility.

As much as the willow tree bends, it always stays true to its roots. The willow does not fly away in the wind or lose its ground. The willow *bends*. What is going on in your life that you are currently standing up strongly to? Could you *bend* a little? I am not saying that we give in to every request, or that we take the path of least resistance each time a challenge presents. What I am saying is that we can learn to *bend* a little in certain situations. Find a little bit of give. Learning to go with the flow in certain situations will help your mind relax and make you a much better person to be around. As we talked about earlier, asking yourself *does it really matter* will help you decide how much you need to bend for each event. If your partner failed to do something they said they would (an all too common argument starter), can you *bend* a little and understand that they may not have wanted to disappoint you – maybe they just had a shit day and it slipped their mind. Maybe you can support them instead of making it worse. Fuel your positive, loving energy instead of a negative, aggressive energy that is only going to hurt both of you. Rewriting your thoughts will play a role in how much you can learn to bend. I must admit that I am still working on my flexibility (both mental and physical), yet every day I know that I am learning to bend a little more, thanks to the story of the willow tree.

STAY IN CONTROL, BY GIVING IT UP

The desire to stay in control relates to one of two things. You either want control because you enjoy the power, or you fear that things will go wrong if you leave it up to someone else. In my case it was for both of those reasons. Being in control is the ultimate illusion of the mind. No one is ever in complete control of anything. Regardless of what we believe, the universe has much more of a say in what happens next than we ever will.

Learning to give up control ties in with what we just talked about in learning to bend like the willow tree. You need to learn to bend and accept that not everything is going to go your way – regardless of whether you are in control or not. Previously I would use 'The Blamer' cognitive distortion and blame anyone or anything for the negative things that occurred in my life. Not only did this make me a victim of circumstances and remove my sense of power over my own destiny, but it also made me want control even more. Subconsciously I would want control because if I controlled everything, it would all go to plan, right? Wrong. This desire for control is nothing but your anxiety wanting you to minimise pain in any form. We need to redesign our mind by rewriting our thoughts to understand that bad things are going to happen no matter who is in control. Counter intuitively, things might actually work out even better if we learn to let go and give up on control, as our grip loosens the pressure of making a mistake.

Are you trying to control what others think about you? You might not directly want to have control, but maybe you are indirectly trying to control or manipulate someone. Maybe you want someone to think of you as a good person and this is why you are so kind to them. Maybe you want validation from them in what they say about you to others. This is another part of your anxiety in that you care too much about what people think. Forget about what anyone says about you. From now on you care about what you say about yourself. You know that if you put in all the right behaviours things will work out – and if someone doesn't like you they must have something wrong with them!

Do you have friends that float through life without having any sense of direction or control over their lives? Maybe they leave it all up to their partner or 'whatever happens, happens'? This is a perfect of example of someone bending like the willow tree, allowing life to happen and accepting the consequences of their actions, whatever they may be. Maybe for us control freaks it would be too much to ask to live life this way, but we can learn something from our friends who seem to float down the river of life. Learning to let go and to forget about trying to control every ship in your harbour will have a massive impact on your mental health. Loosen your grip on life, bend a little and watch this part of your anxiety reduce dramatically. Know that voluntarily giving up control is the ultimate way to have control over your own mind.

BE AVERAGE YOU PERFECTIONIST WANKER

Are you a perfectionist? Do you strive to keep things perfect just as I used to? As I am sure you know by now, nothing in life is perfect. By setting perfectionist standards for ourselves and others, we are causing unnecessary stress in our lives. I believe that the quest for perfect is just anxiety in disguise. We are only trying to make things perfect due to the fear of getting it wrong.

I now ask myself what the costs and benefits are of being a perfectionist. The benefits are that things will go right most of the time due to your attention to detail, and you will spend little time fixing up mistakes. You will probably feel good about yourself most of the time for being 'perfect'. However, there is always a cost. Stress, anxiety, worry, disappointment (when you actually do stuff something up), nervousness, pressure and grey hairs are some of the costs. Studies also show that high blood pressure, high cholesterol, obesity, early ageing and even heart attacks can be caused by stress. Being on edge constantly has some good points but do you want to be a perfectionist and suffer the consequences? This all ties in with wanting to maintain control, and just to remind you again, having control does not mean that things won't go wrong. Being a perfectionist does not mean that you won't make mistakes. The ultimate shackle of being a perfectionist is that no matter how good you have been so far, you are only happy with what happens next.

You might not even think you are a perfectionist. Do you want the perfect partner? Do you want your work to be the best? Do you have high standards for your kids? Are you a clean freak? Do you get frustrated when you make a mistake? Do you fear living a few days with an unread inbox? Do you expect friends and family to hold themselves to your high standards too? These are all ways of the perfectionist. Think about one of your less perfectionist friends. You know, the one who doesn't give a shit? Is he or she a perfectionist? No way! Are they happy? More than likely. They still put effort into things but are unfazed as to whether they turn out 'perfectly' or not. Learning not to be a perfectionist is a great way to release control and anxiety from your life. You might actually do better once you loosen your grip on a situation and move freely without the fear of failure.

Even the model on the front page of a magazine has something 'imperfect' about her. Look around the room you are sitting in. Is something out of place? Is there a small mark on a wall that you never noticed before? What about the world we live in? Are the beaches perfectly square? Are the mountain's perfectly symmetrical? Is the grass all the same shade of green? Nothing is perfect! Surprisingly, even this book is not perfect! Redesign Your Mind has been *redesigned* many times and yet it is still not perfect. Could it be better? Of course. Could it be worse? Of course. Will it help people? Yes! I could have sat here *redesigning* this book for years in a quest for perfection. Would it really have mattered? I don't think so. I am a writer who is vulnerable and *average* just like the rest of you? I know that when I was going through challenges with anxiety and depression I just wanted to know that there was someone like me who has faced the same challenge. Maybe the perfectionists who read this book can find a way to loosen up in the quest of being perfectly *average*? Do some thinking and decide whether being a perfectionist is adding to your happiness or not. Once you know what is important to you, rewrite your thoughts again and again until you are no longer perfect.

WRITE A JOURNAL

We know that rewriting our thoughts is an invaluable practice in the designing of our mind. We can add another layer to our practice with the writing of a journal. This will be similar yet different to rewriting your thoughts. You can decide how you would like to write your journal. Some people find that writing a daily log of what happened in their day is a great way to let out any negative emotions and move on to the next day, while others find that writing about only certain topics helps best. I have tried both of these methods and found that while living a busy life it was best to do a weekly summary journal. Remember that you will have to dedicate time to rewriting your thoughts, so maybe you can practice writing a journal less frequently. You can write about anything in your journal. Maybe you will write about your redesigning your mind journey.

As my thoughts started to change due to rewriting them day in, day out, I found that writing a weekly summary was a good way to reflect. As you get stronger and stronger, you might find that you fill out your journal once a month instead – but I will leave this up to you. Below is the method I used for my journal to help me reflect on what I achieved in the last week and set mini-goals for the week ahead. I sit down for just 10 minutes and write out the following;

THE WEEKLY JOURNAL
What did I achieve this week, and / or what did I do for the first time?
What would I like to challenge myself to change or improve on next week?
What is something that I am doing well that I will keep doing?
How am I going with the most important things in my life?

Writing this journal will help plant your goals for self-improvement into your subconscious and give you positive vibes for the things you have achieved. Often we overlook how far we have come, and by writing out this journal you will now stop and think about all the good things you have done. Try and keep it to just a few dot points on each section. You will feel amazed by what you are achieving, empowered for challenging yourself, and constructive for what you are already doing well. The journal will help you to be mindful of what you want to achieve and hold you accountable for the things you said you would do but haven't. It will serve as a reminder that there still may be work for you to do.

Each time you write in your journal, I want you to go back to what you wrote last time and see how you are going. Are you still doing the things that you said you would keep doing? Did you follow through with the things that you would like to challenge yourself with? You can even put little ticks next to things once you know you have achieved them (ticks will make you feel good). Put a star next to anything that you still need to work on. How are you going with the most important things in your life? Are they still even important? Have you since redesigned what is important to you and now need to adjust? Flicking back through my journal and seeing some of the things I wrote only a few years ago really was a powerful moment for me. It proved how far I had come, and also how far I have to go. Your journal will be something you can be proud of. It is a part of you and a reflection of your ever-changing new mindset.

BREATHE

In the game of life you breathe or you die. I am sure that everyone reading this book is still breathing (call a doctor if not), however the thing is that we often do not breathe properly. Without even knowing, my breathing was having a massive effect on my mental health. Through a guided meditation with my psychologist (personal trainer for the mind), I learnt that I am a shallow breather. This means that although I take in oxygen when I breathe in, often I am not breathing in deeply. My breath is not going in all the way down to my diaphragm which means that I am not getting the full benefit of the air that I breathe. When an anxious moment comes along, you can guess what happens to my breath. It gets faster and shorter, as if my body is preparing itself for battle. This response is known as the flight or fight response. This bodily symptom of anxiety is something that we can easily learn to control just by paying attention to it.

To find out if you are breathing deeply or not, sit on a chair and put your fingers over your diaphragm region. Have the fingers from your left and right hand barely touching together over your diaphragm. Breathe in and watch your fingers move apart (and back together) as you breathe in and out. This means that you are now breathing in deeply. This is how we want to breathe. When we are breathing in too shallowly, our fingers wouldn't move out as much and it means that we are preparing for the fight or flight.

I know it might sound silly but breathing properly is something we forget to do when we are tight and tense. We can help train our mind and body to breathe in properly by paying attention to our breath. To help you remember to practice breathing deeply, put a little reminder in your phone, on your computer or on a sticky note. The more you practice, the more you will notice yourself sitting there and paying attention to your breath. You will start to tune into when you are getting anxious, realising that your breathing has become shallow and you need to deepen your breath. Slowing your breath down by counting to three on the way in and out will also help. Actively checking in with your breathing forms part of your mindfulness. Search on YouTube for a few videos on the effect of the breath and different breathing techniques to help you on your journey. Check in with your breath when you notice that you are becoming anxious and make it a habit to breathe in a little deeper and a little slower. Knowing how your breath is going and what you can do to change it will help you take control of your body when anxiety leading events come about. Use your breath to your advantage in the quest to redesign your mind.

SUMMARISE THE DAY

This is one of my personal favourites. Do you ever come home after a tough day at work and bombard your partner, or whoever is in the house at the time, with all your problems? We have all been there. I used to spend much of my time talking with family about the negative parts of my day. Little time would be spent on anything good. This is a negatively fuelled way to spend our time. Not only are those shit parts of the day already over and not related to what we are doing with our family at night, but by continuously talking about them we encourage and inflate the negative thoughts which bring on our negative emotions. We are attracting a negative vibe and whoever we are talking to wouldn't be happy about the conversation they just had (even if they don't know it). We only have so much free time in a day, so why waste most of it talking about the negative parts of the day? Summarising the day is a great way to help us acknowledge (and move on) from some of the challenges we face in a day, allowing time for the best parts and things we are looking forward to tomorrow.

I know that we still need to get these things off of our chest; however, we can do it in a way that is effective, efficient, and then allows us to move on without repetition. Something that I experimented with my family was to have a '5-minute summary of our day' for each person in the family. I was amazed by how effective this was in changing our energy and how we spent our time together. An important part of the process is not to complain about your day or any challenges outside of this 5-minute window. Before talking about anything else from your day, you sit down together and spend 5 minutes each on the following;

5 MINUTE SUMMARY OF THE DAY
What was the best part of your day?
What was the most challenging (*instead of saying worst!*) part of your day?
What is something that happened today that made you laugh?
What is something that you are looking forward to tomorrow?

You will be amazed by the conversations you are going to have and how much of a positive spin this will put on the end of your day. Set a timer on your phone for 5 minutes per person; meaning that if there are two of you it will take 10 minutes total. I was amazed at how many laughs we were having and how the challenges were condensed to only a few short minutes – freeing up more time to talk about the good things.

I have structured the questions in this manner because our minds remember the most about the first or last thing that was said in a particular conversation. By starting the conversation with the best part of your day, and ending with something that you are looking forward to, you are starting and ending with the positive. Oh yeah, and after this conversation is done, that's it. No more complaining about the boss at work or something that annoyed you. If you have a genuine challenge that is going to need to be worked through then I suggest sitting down and writing out your thoughts and working through the problem. Sure you can ask for other people's opinions, but if it is something that can wait – maybe write it down and come back to it next week. A week later it probably won't even be an issue in your life anymore. If it is just something that happened and there is no further action required or decisions that need to be made, then you leave it there and move on to enjoying the rest of your spare time.

My mind was now redesigned as I found that during the day I would be looking for the best parts, the shit parts and the funny parts – ready to present to the group that night. This made the day much more enjoyable as I was no longer focusing on just the negative events that occurred and I could actively pursue the best and funny parts too. I also found that it was a fun way to get all the family together and share a good time. If someone is having a challenging time, the laughs and smiles from the rest of the group can help them forget about this challenge for a few minutes. Let's compare this to the family where someone comes home after having a shit day and they spend twenty minutes water boarding you about it. After this time you most likely want to get out of the room. You have no interest in discussing the good parts of the day. I doubt there will be any room for laughter or what you are looking forward to tomorrow. Learn to summarise the day and watch how your happiness, laughter and positive outlook for the future grows with each nightly conversation.

CHAPTER TEN
REDESIGN YOUR PERSPECTIVE

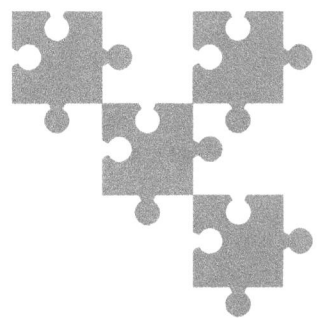

CREATE YOUR OWN MEANING OF LIFE

The meaning of life is a big question that remains unanswered to this day. It is fine that we don't know the answer; however an existential crisis is going to cultivate depressive-causing thoughts about the lack of explicitness around the meaning of life. I used to search for a clear reason as to what I *should* do with my life, particularly during times of depression or uncertainty. Unfortunately I don't believe that I will find this clarity in my lifetime as we are yet to find the magical stone on which the meaning of life was written. One thing I do believe is that if there was a meaning of life, 20,000 years ago the meaning would have been very different to 100 years ago, and 100 years ago it would have been very different to today. Society and technology have greatly changed what the 'meaning of life' is for us compared to our ancestors. I imagine that if robots take over most of the tasks in our lives in another 100 years' time, our meaning will look very different again. 20,000 years ago the meaning may have been 'just to survive' and now it may be seen by society as 'to thrive'.

Why are we on a continual quest for the meaning of life when we could be creating our own meaning? You are the one who is going to have to get out of bed every morning. You are the one who is going to have to go to work and pay bills. You are the one who is going to need to find a reason for you, by you, to make this all happen. Deep down you might actually know your meaning already, but you just can't find it. This book might help you find it. Once we find our meaning we need to do everything within our power to live the life that fulfils this meaning. If you don't actively make a choice to make this happen, then you are wasting your time. You are using your energy for nothing other than a purpose that is not yours. This is definitely not the meaning of life and something I want you to move away from. I was fulfilling a meaning that was not mine, and now that I have found *my* meaning I couldn't be happier. For me, my meaning of life revolves around fulfilling my purpose to make this world a better place. Not just for my family, but for many more. I want to have fun doing it too. How I serve this life meaning may change as time goes on, but for now I am happy doing what I am doing. My path might change in the future but the purpose I am serving will always remain.

Everything I do is fulfilling this purpose in some way. Exercise doesn't seem like I am making the world a better place or having fun – but it is giving me strength to keep going when times get tough. It improves my flexibility, physical and mental health. This is part of my meaning and helps me to go on when things get tough in yoga class and I want to go home. My job might not seem like it is my life's meaning, but earning an income to help fund my lifestyle, and my book is part of my meaning. These examples will help you understand that there are things that we need but may not want to do to help us fulfil our life's meaning.

Man's Search for Meaning by Viktor E. Frankl will help you understand that we can put up with unimaginable challenges if we have meaning. If there is a reason to get through the pain, you will find a way. Since no one else has ever given us an official meaning of life, I am giving you permission to write your own meaning. Create a meaning that is for you. A life motto. A reason why you are here. Write it down, put it on the wall and put it in your heart. If this meaning is true, then rewriting your thoughts and getting your life on the path that you want it to be on will be the easiest thing you ever done.

ACT AS IF

'Act As If' is a powerful saying that will help you in times of uncertainty. I would love to say that 'Act as if' came from a respected philosopher but embarrassingly I learnt 'Act as if' from a speech Ben Affleck gave in the Hollywood film *Boiler Room*. If you have seen this movie, you would know that the character who delivers this speech is an arrogant dick who rips people off to get rich. Yes, this is not the behaviour we want to model ourselves on; however his way of building confidence for the short term is something we can all apply in our lives.

'Act as if' means that in any situation, you can 'act as if' you are someone else or 'act as if' you are feeling an emotion different to the one you are feeling now. Putting this façade or layer on is empowering during situations when you feel as if your power to keep cool may be taken away. We still need to work on rewriting our thoughts to help us remove these anxious or depressive-leading thoughts, but for the short term using 'act as if' will help you from having any major setbacks. In my own life I know that I often perform better when I feel like I have nothing to lose. 'Acting as if' I have nothing to lose releases the pressure in a situation and helps me to decide and act freely without the fear of losing what I have already got. That is just how I best use 'act as if' but here are a few more examples on how you can use it.

ACT AS IF EXAMPLES	
SCENARIO	ACT AS IF RESPONSE
1. You walk into a room and feel anxious about everyone looking at you 2. You are nervous about a big exam 3. You are scared to lose someone. 4. You are worried about what someone is saying about you 5. You are depressed as you do not like your job	1. 'Act as if' you are a famous celebrity. Everyone wants to be your friend. 2. 'Act as if' you already passed OR 'Act as if' it doesn't matter. 3. 'Act as if' you never had them OR 'Act as if' they are not yours to lose OR 'Act as if you will always remember the good times without fear of not seeing them again. 4. 'Act as if' you don't care what they say about you OR 'Act as if' you agree with what they are saying about you 5. 'Act as if' you are happy that you realised you need to change OR 'act as if' you are just in this job temporarily until you find a better one OR 'act as if you enjoy certain parts of the job'

You will have your own scenarios where you can 'act as if'. Remember that this is just a temporary solution to short circuit moments of anxiety or depression. It is best used in situations when you feel a wave of anxiety or depression and you need something to help you get through the moment. Going home and rewriting your thoughts is going to help you understand *why* you have these flashes of anxiety or depression and then work through them by redesigning your mind to reduce their impact in the future. 'Act as if' is your safety net for anything in the short term.

PROCESS V OUTCOME

Have you ever executed something well and according to plan but it still turned to shit? We can laugh now but at the time it really hurts. We know that shit happens in life but why do we get so worked up when the shit actually hits the fan? The reason is because we are too focused on the *outcome* and not the *process*. The outcome is exactly that – how things turned out. The process is the behaviours and practices we put in place to make it all happen. What we need to learn to separate is those moments when we did everything right, and the moments we didn't actually put all the right behaviours and practices in place. Maybe there are times where we are using 'The Blamer' cognitive distortion and putting our shortcomings on to someone else. Maybe there are times where we can take more responsibility for what happened. I bet you would be surprised and maybe a little defensive to hear that I don't think there would be many times where we weren't the slightest bit responsible for an event not going to plan – even though we don't like to admit it.

By learning to use the 'process v outcome' tool, we can actually identify when we were responsible for something going wrong and when *shit happens*. If we were responsible even in the slightest bit, we can learn from this event and do things differently next time. This empowers us to use this experience as a building block to become a better person instead of feeling powerless and bringing on the negative emotions that come with it. If we couldn't have done anything differently, and it was only due to unforeseen circumstances that something went wrong, we can shrug our shoulders and say 'that's life'. We did everything we could and we don't need to change anything for next time. Two candidates may go for a job and do everything within their power to get it, yet only one of them will be chosen. This is out of our control and as talked about earlier, this is something we cannot allow to get to us. Here is how I use the process v outcome tool. Use it whenever you need to learn from an event in your life, helping yourself move on and grow from the experience.

> **PROCESS V OUTCOME TOOL**
>
> 1. **Did something go wrong?**
> If YES > keep going
> 2. **Did I make any mistakes?**
> If YES > write down your mistakes and learn from them
> If NO > keep going
> 3. **Was there anything I could have done better or differently?**
> If YES > write down the things you could have done better or differently and learn from them
> If NO > keep going
> 4. **Was there anything in my control I could have done to change this outcome?**
> If Yes > write down the things that were in your control that you could have done. Do these things next time
> If NO > Shit happens. You have done everything you could have done and the outcome was out of your control. Write down some inspiring, positive thoughts and try again next time.

It seems so simple doesn't it? If only we had this tool when we were younger we could have saved ourselves a lot of heartache and learnt from a lot of our mistakes. Just like all the other tools in this book, it will only work if you use it. By using this tool each time something goes wrong you will work through the problem instead of just replaying the negative thoughts about how the outcome was not what you wanted. Most of the times you will find that you had a role to play in this outcome and you can learn from it for next time. This gives you the power back and helps you move on. And move on you will to the successful redesign of your mind.

CHAPTER ELEVEN
REDESIGNING LIFE

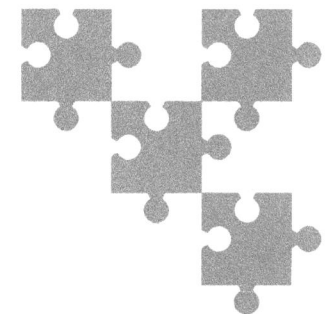

REDESIGN YOUR RELATIONSHIPS

Relationships are one of the biggest yet most rewarding challenges we face in our lives. Whether it is a relationship with a partner, your family, friends or colleagues at work, your relationships and how you treat other people are important contributors to your mental health. For most of this book we are working on the redesign of your mind; however we need to understand that those around us will also have influence on how we feel. One of the challenges we face with relationships in this day and age is that we have so many of them. Technology and social media have made it easier than ever to keep in touch with multiple people from all over the world, all at the same time. Whilst this is a beautiful thing, it also provides its challenges.

Trying to maintain several relationships not only requires a lot of time and energy but can also limit the depth of each relationship we have. It's not hard to work out that if you have X amount of time to devote to relationships with others, that if you have more people to split that time between, you are not going to be able to cultivate that same connection with each person. In terms of finding a partner, this makes it extremely challenging as we often have little time to judge whether a candidate is suitable or not. Apps like Tinder and Bumble have programmed our minds to think that a relationship is based on someone's looks, what exotic holidays they have been on and whether they have a dog or not. There is no time to cultivate a connection because before we know it there is someone or something else on the scene to grab our attention. We have never been in such a connected world, yet we fail to *connect*.

Basing our happiness on our relationship status or how our relationship is going is totally removing the power of our happiness from ourselves. Just as we talked about in earlier sections, a relationship is largely out of our control. There are two (or more if you are adventurous) people in a relationship. We can seek a relationship and use tools such as 'Process v Outcome' to determine if there is anything that we can change to help the process – otherwise we can accept that we have to keep doing what we are doing and hope that the right person will come along. Are you doing everything in your power to help find a partner? Are you looking your best? Are you going out to the right places? Are you your fittest? Are you giving people a go? Have you redesigned your mind? Are you giving off the right energy? Are you saying that you want a relationship but your actions tell a different story? These are all questions you need to answer for yourself and get to work on how you can make this happen. Forget about the lucky stories you hear from your friends. Maybe you will get lucky too. Maybe you can do everything within your power to try and find someone and leave the *outcome* up to the universe.

Whether it is a potential partner or a new friend, you need to do everything you can to create and maintain the relationship. I mentioned that we need to give people a go, but this is something we are not genuinely doing. Are you perfect? Of course not! So why do we expect someone else to be perfect? Why are we ruling out the possibilities of something amazing by not giving them a chance? What has this book told you about 'acting as if' and 'redesigning your mind' and 'creating the life that you want to live'? How can you create this life without taking a chance on someone? Take responsibility and redesign your relationships. Maybe you can get help from a psychologist (personal trainer for the mind). There is nothing stopping you from redesigning how you behave, act and contribute to a relationship. Tell your partner what *you* are going to do to make this work. You don't want or need them to change. Instead *you* will change and become better. If the outcome of the relationship is not what you want, then move on. You have a lot to give to someone, and if the values, beliefs and actions of your partner or friends do not match yours, then maybe it is a time for a change of environment. Yes, it is sad, but so is spending the rest of your life with people that are not right for you.

There may have been some tough words in that last section but I hope you got something out of it. You are in control of your life and it is up to you to *decide* how you want to live it. You are the one who is going to have to live it. Not me and not one of your friends. Take responsibility for who you want to be and get to work on making it happen. The way you treat other people might also need to change. Just as we are cultivating a new mindset and redesigning the way we live our life, we may need to redesign how we speak to others. This involves how we treat others and what we expect from another person. Give people the benefit of the doubt. Love them for who they are. Speak to them as if they are special to you. The most valuable thing we can get out of life comes from our relationships. Love and friendship wouldn't exist if you lived in a world by yourself. Yeah, sure, you could drive all the hottest cars, wear all the best clothes and eat the finest foods – but it wouldn't mean shit if you didn't have someone to share it with. Show immense love for your partner, family, friends and anyone else around you because at the end of the day they will be the most valuable possessions you will ever have.

MONEY, MONEY, MONEY

Who likes money? I know I do. Before I *redesigned my mind*, much of my life was driven by money. Making it and wishing that I had more of it took up much of my time. When I was younger I always thought that by age 30 I would be rich and writing a book on how to become rich. Its funny how at that exact age of 30, I am now writing a book on how to redesign your mind and forget about things like money. Society has conditioned us to want and *need* more money. The capitalist world we live in is all about earning and spending money. Commercials and advertisements are all about attracting your money, starting in our most formative years as a child. Lotteries and our perception of the rich condition us to want large amounts of money instead of large amounts of love. We grow up thinking we need more money and more stuff to be happy. It is time to redesign what money means to us.

If you are like me, you need to add into the process of rewriting your thoughts that 'no amount of money will make you happy'. I agree that even a small part of me still thinks, *hmm if I had ten million dollars I am sure I would be happie*r – but it no longer consumes my goals or defines what it mean to be 'successful'. We talked about redefining what success and ambition means to you. Money is most likely only going to be a small part of what brings you happiness.

I know that some of you will still think that money can bring you ultimate happiness. You are reading this while laughing. I would be too. The fact is that money is scientifically proven not to bring you happiness. Money.com wrote about a study that took in results from 1.7 million people over 164 different countries to determine the sweet spot of money and happiness. The study found that people are happiest on an income of around $75,000 per year (Ducharme, 2018). Is this not an amazing figure? Even more surprising is that one of the studies showed that people actually had a decline in emotional well-being and life satisfaction when earning over $95,000 per year. How is this even possible?

We spend so much of our lives chasing higher incomes, more money, bigger houses and flashier toys yet the research shows that our happiness is basically at its highest when we earn $75,000 per year, per person.

I know that some of you *still* don't believe me. You think you are different and that if you could just have that little bit extra that everything would be oh so much better. This is one part of your mind that you will need to redesign. You need to understand that the illusion with money is that you always want more. That is it. Money is a never-ending cycle that involves chasing and chasing until you die. There will always be a new toy, a bigger house, another holiday or children to provide for. This is the ultimate illusion that our society has created. Before the creation of money there was nothing that we would chase. We lived off the land and stocking up on things wasn't possible. Animals roamed free and you couldn't stock up on meat in the freezer. There was nothing to buy with money. We have created money and in it we have created a never-ending chase.

Let's look at the rich. Why don't the rich stop chasing money once they reach a certain amount? Why aren't the rich driving around in their flashy cars with bigger smiles on their faces? It is all because money doesn't 'buy' happiness. The rich have problems just like us. Yes, it is nice to turn up to your problems in a Porsche instead of a beat-up piece of crap, just like Jordan Belfort states in *The Wolf of Wall Street*, but his problems ended up costing him a fortune and resulted in a great amount of pain for his family. I love *The Wolf of Wall Street*, but I don't think turning up to those problems in a Porsche would make a difference.

Research and the lack of rich people singing songs of joy all day prove that money does not buy happiness – and too much of it will make you worse off. Biggie said it best with *Mo Money, Mo Problems*. I have worked in finance for most of my working life and I can tell you that it is not about how much money you make, it is all about what you do with it. If you live outside of your means and try to keep up with the Jones' then you are never going to have enough. If you spend less than you earn and save some of your money, then things are going to work out. Find other things to bring you happiness instead of money. When all the research shows that money does not buy you happiness, why make yourself a slave to it? If there was something, anything that told us otherwise then I would allow it but as we talked about in earlier sections, your happiness is going to come from your mindset, your energy, your relationships and finding meaning in your life. If you *still* don't believe that money doesn't matter, ask yourself one of these questions. Has anyone close to you ever died?

Who is the person you care most about in the world? If you had a magical genie who offered you the choice of a million dollars or this person's life for the rest of your days – which would you chose? Money doesn't mean shit.

DESIGN YOUR HEADSTONE

Have you ever thought about how you want to be remembered? One of the characters in the movie *Seven Days in Utopia* asks, 'What do you want written on your headstone?' This is a powerful question that brought out deep emotions when I first watched it. I asked myself this question during the redesign of my mind. We have talked about money and 'success'. Do you want your headstone to say 'Jenny died with $9,250,714 in her bank account'? Maybe 'Jenny died with 400,000 Instagram followers'? I don't think this is how anyone wants to be remembered and unfortunately this is one of the reasons why we have so much anxiety and depression in the world we live in today. We chase a goal that has no meaning. We chase money that has no value. We chase someone else's dream.

Today is the day that you no longer chase what is important to someone else. This is the moment when you decide what is important to you and go about living the life that is going to fulfil your happiness. Think about what you want written on your headstone because this is another way of connecting with your higher self. The answer helps guide you toward the type of person you want to be. Deciding what I want to be written on my tombstone truly helped inspire me to redesign my mind. I hope it will help you change perspective and cultivate a mindset that chases real goals and real meaning.

CHAPTER TWELVE
ROADBLOCKS TO YOUR HAPPINESS

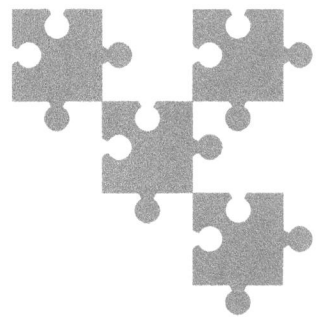

OH SHIT, THAT DIDN'T WORK

I want you to know that I have tried many things on the journey to redesigning my mind. I have spent years of research, practice and self-development to find what works for me and my happiness. One thing I know is that there are a lot of things that don't work. I also found that some of the things that worked for someone else didn't work for me. You might find some of the tools and practices in this book invaluable to redesigning of your mind whilst some of them less so. That is ok because you are on a journey of finding out what works best for you.

Redesigning your mind is about constant change. You might find that something that didn't work for you today will work for you tomorrow. Don't be scared to try something again. What is not ok is giving up and saying that you are just going to accept that 'this is the way I am'. By now you have learnt that we have the capacity to change and to grow. No matter how hard you have tried without success, or how hard you have worked on something, never give up. Keep trying until you find something that works for you. I know that if you implement a lot of the changes discussed in this book you will go a long way to being the person you want to be. It is time to go through some of the potential roadblocks that will get in the way of your new mindset. Look out for these roadblocks and do your best to work through them.

FINDING WAYS TO ESCAPE THE PAIN

Like any young person, it was easy to find a way to mask my problems. During my times of not accepting my anxiety and depression, I would turn to alcohol, illicit substances, random sex, gambling and anything else that took my mind off the worry and pain for a short while. Whilst these things made me feel good at the time, I can tell you that in the long run they all made things much worse. Alcohol and any kind of illicit or abused substance will just make your reality that much harder when you wake up depressed and hung-over. Random sex was just a way to validate myself as still being worthy which left me feeling empty and lonely when it was all done. Gambling was just a way to try and win enough money to buy me back my happiness. No matter how much I won, I could never buy myself out of trouble. Whilst I dabbled with these behaviours, I was 'lucky' that I did not fall into an addiction. If this is you, get the help that you need to put this self-destructive behaviour behind you. Sure it is great to still have fun, but this is a good time to ask yourself whether you are having fun or just trying to escape a reality. If you believe that these behaviours are just ways to try and escape your reality, then you need to take action and find a new way to bring back your happiness.

REDESIGNING DISAPPOINTMENT

Disappointment comes from expectation. If you removed expectation you would never be disappointed. I still get disappointed from time to time, but by rewriting my thoughts I notice how much of my disappointment was brought on by expectations that I set. Remember that we cannot control external environments. All we can control is our processes and how we react when shit happens. Are you setting unnecessary expectations? Are you holding yourself or someone else to high standards? Are you expecting things to go magically well after you finish reading this book? All of these expectations are setting you up for disappointment if the outcome is not as you planned.

It is ok to feel a little disappointed from time to time but look into the reasons why you are disappointed and learn from them. Is this something you can learn from or was there nothing you could do about it? Don't beat yourself up over any negative outcome. You can be constructively disappointed but use this emotion to help drive your improvement and self-development. It is up to you to decide how you are going to use disappointment in your life. From this day forward it can continue to leave you feeling depressed, or it can fuel a hunger and desire to do better next time.

DISEASE

Many of the motivational speakers, such as Tony Robbins, talk about disease and phrase the word as two separate portions being dis-ease. Dis-ease is when you are not at ease and potentially in pain. We put our bodies and minds through so much pain when we have a dis-ease in the mind. Negative thoughts and an uncertainty on how to remove this dis-ease are a massive reason why people stay in this position for so long. I put myself through so much suffering due to my dis-ease. Physical symptoms appeared when there was nothing wrong with my body. Headaches, a stiff neck, heart palpitations, nausea, upset stomachs, shaking, dizziness, poor vision, sore throats and tiredness are all some of the psychosomatic symptoms I experienced in my battle with mental illness.

Eventually I accepted that my symptoms were from a dis-eased mind and nothing else. These physical symptoms are a roadblock to your happiness. You will use 'The Blamer' cognitive distortion to give excuses as to why you cannot beat anxiety or depression. You will distract yourself with physical symptoms and reason why you can't be happy. This is all the defence of your old mind, fighting for its right to hold its power over you so that you don't have to do the hard work to redesign your mind. You need to take charge of your mindset by rewriting your thoughts and working on your meaning, your environment and what type of person you want to be. I promise you that as you take this power back and continue to work on your life, these psychosomatic symptoms will release their hold over you.

Get to work on your new life and free yourself from the dis-ease of the past. Don't be scared to challenge your mind and challenge yourself to push on when things get tough. Sure, you will be tired and would rather watch TV instead of rewriting your thoughts, but you need to understand that making this decision to take action instead of letting it slide will be a massive step forward in curing your dis-ease and stopping you from feeling sorry for yourself.

OVERWHELM

Overwhelm is all about stress. You fear there is too much to do and you might not get it all done. You fear the consequences that your actions today may have in the future. Just like the rest of the negative emotions we feel, overwhelm only exists in our mind. Overwhelm is our personal alert system preparing us for the 'fight or flight' response. It is our mind telling us that there is a lot to do. It may also be that our mind is so overloaded with thought that it can no longer function properly. You have overloaded your system and you need to give it time to cool.

How can we reduce the overwhelming feeling when things get tough? You can meditate and practice mindfulness to help you get through the immediate short term feeling of being overwhelmed; however, in the long term, you need to work on deeper reasons why you are overwhelmed. This goes back to the change of mindset or change of environment. Are you in an environment that is too hot to handle? This could be working in a job that stresses you out. It could be living with your family who all expect too much of you. It is up to you to help create the environment that you want.

Maybe it is a change of mindset that you need. Maybe you need to rewrite your thoughts to help cultivate a mindset that says you are ok with things not being complete all the time. The Daoist say that 'if nothing is done, then nothing is undone'. Can we choose to leave things undone? Has it just been our mind that is creating pressure on us to have all the boxes ticked and everything ready by a certain time? Can we ask ourselves *does it really matter?* I have practiced this in my own life and found that most of the overwhelming feelings I experience are a result of my own mind. No one else put that pressure on me. Learning to relieve yourself of this pressure that you put onto yourself by rewriting your thoughts will help you go a long way to removing overwhelm.

WAITING TO BE HAPPY

I found that I always had a reason to delay my happiness, as if I were waiting for something to happen before I could allow myself to be happy. This can go on and on until you realise that you have waited your whole life to be happy without enjoying the journey. The journey, not the destination, is the reward. It is awesome to have goals and dreams, but to hinge our happiness on waiting for something that may not even happen is just bizarre. This living in the future creates anxious emotions, and eventually sets us up for depression if these things don't happen.

Stop waiting for things to happen before you can be happy. If there is something that you want to do (*like writing a book for example*), don't wait for someone to offer you a contract to start writing, or for you to get more experience, or to become wiser; just *start writing*. And then don't hinge your happiness on whether the book is a success or not. These negative thoughts keep you from enjoying yourself in the present moment and lead to depressed, anxious, emotive states. Instead enjoy the journey of writing the book because it is something you want to do. This creates a positive, carefree mindset as opposed to the anxiety and depressive, expectation driven thoughts of waiting for happiness. Keeping our life in balance means our happiness does not depend on one area of our life. If writing a book is a flop then you will have something to laugh about over a few drinks with your friends.

No longer will we spend any energy on what other people think. Instead we will focus our attention on the things that we actually give a f*ck about. Sure, things are going to fall out of whack from time to time but being self-aware is going to help you bring things back into line. Choose where you want to spend your time and energy wisely – because there is no point having a million dollars in the bank if you are not happy. Acknowledge that you can be happy right here and now with whatever it is that you already have in your life. Yes, we can strive for more but ultimately we don't need to achieve anything more to be happy.

TALKING TO EVERYONE ABOUT YOUR PROBLEMS

When I was at my lowest low, well before I started reading books about the mind and getting help from my psychologist (personal trainer for the mind); I would ask anyone and everyone how they would deal with my problems. I would seek validation that my problems were real problems and hope that they would have an answer for me. Unfortunately many of the people didn't have anything useful to contribute other than to 'not worry about it' or that it was 'just a rough patch, you'll be fine'. I eventually noticed that I was having the same conversation – just with different people. This was a major roadblock. My mind was just trying to waste time and keep me down by replaying the same discussions over and over again.

Eventually I learnt that talking about my problems was great at first. It felt good to get it off my chest. However, it was no longer helping me move forward. Whilst I am a massive advocate for talking to someone and getting help, I am also a believer that we need to talk about working on our problems and taking action to move forward – not just replay the same conversations about why it is so much harder for you. The challenge for our society is to learn to move forward with our problems and find solutions, not just talk about them.

LOCKING YOURSELF AWAY

I may have mentioned earlier how I locked myself away from most of my friends and social activities while I was in the dumps. I really shut myself off and whilst I thought it was good at the time, I now would have done this differently. Life is all about balance, and I know you may have a lot of work to do on the redesign of your mind. The thing is that a balanced lifestyle is going to help our mental health more than anything. How things are balanced is up to you, but it is important that you continue to spend time with friends and make social appearances while you are making this all happen.

Learning to feel comfortable with ourselves and where we are in life gives us the power over the fact that we are not going to let anxiety, depression or the need for a new mindset stop us from living our life. Use tools such as 'Act as If' to help release the pressure. With less pressure to want to be someone else, you will allow yourself time to heal, time to grow, and time to redesign your mind.

CHAPTER THIRTEEN
REDESIGN YOUR LUCK

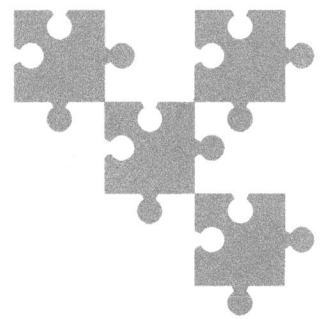

THE OLD MAN AT THE FORT

I love a good story. One that stands out in my mind is *The Old Man at the Fort* which I read in *The Importance of Living* by Lin Yutang. Society has conditioned us to think that we are either lucky or unlucky, often influencing how we feel about life. In certain situations we are quick to label ourselves 'lucky' or 'unlucky' without taking the time to stop and think about the long term implications of this so called 'luck'. The story of *The Old Man at the Fort* helped me understand that we do not need to jump to conclusions (cognitive distortion) on many of the situations in our lives. I hope this story helps you in the same way it helped me. Just as it did for me, I know this story will help you on your journey of self-development. Here is my impression of *The Old Man at the Fort*.

Many years ago there was an old man who lived with his son on the family farm. They had one horse and one day the gate was left open and the horse ran away. The neighbours came around a few days later and said, 'Oh no, that is bad luck you have lost your horse'. The old man asked the neighbour if it was good luck or bad luck. How do we know? A few months later the horse returned, and with it came another four horses that followed it from the wild. The neighbours visited a few days later and said, 'Oh, you are so lucky you have four horses; now I wish I was as lucky as you'. The old man then asked the neighbours whether it was really good luck or not. How do we know if it is good luck? Now that the old man had more than one horse he was able to go riding on horseback together with his son. One day his son fell off and broke his back, instantly labelled as a cripple. The doctors confirmed that the son would never walk again and would be confined to his home for the rest of his life. The neighbours came around and with much disappointment said, 'we are so sorry that you have such bad luck; your son's life is ruined'. The old man's beliefs must have been tested. The old man could have lost all hope and replied with something negative; yet as usual he replied, 'how do we know if this is good luck or bad luck? *I'm sure that by this stage the neighbours would have felt like this old man was delusional.*

The old man continued to care for his son. A few years later the army marched into town and ordered that all men of age were to be sent to war. The old man would just slow them down and was not required. His son was of the right age; however the army said that they didn't want to take the 'cripple' as he would be too much of a burden. So the 'unlucky' cripple stayed home with his father while all the 'lucky' men marched off to war. A few weeks later word reached town that the men who went to war were caught up in a battle. There were no survivors. The old man was now forever grateful for what happened to his 'unlucky' son, enjoying the rest of his days in the comfort of their home.

Now tell me who was unlucky and who was lucky in that story? I am sure at different stages of the story you would have changed your mind! This is a powerful demonstration of how we cannot look at things right away and label them as 'good' or 'bad' or 'lucky' or 'unlucky'. This story gives you hope when it would be so easy to conclude that there is none. Relating this to my own life, I can look at experiencing anxiety and depression in my 20's as good luck or bad luck. Yes, it was a challenging time, and yes, there was much pain and suffering throughout. However, we can say that now that I have redesigned my mind and redesigned my life, I couldn't be happier.

We all have the ultimate luck in that we won a big race to even be conceived and be born. Your experience of consciousness and life is something that is chosen for a limited few. There couldn't be a better time to be alive and it is up to us to look for the positives in a situation, or at least wait to see if a negative event actually turns out to be a 'lucky' one.

PROS AND CONS

Every pro has a con and every con has a pro. Life is a double-edged sword in that when good things happen, there is also a loss or 'cost' and vice versa. Just like the story of the Chinese Farmer, we can acknowledge that what might not seem like a positive event in the short term, may actually turn out to be the best thing that has ever happened to us. There is always a silver lining. Take these examples

Event > you start a new relationship

Pro > you are extremely happy with your new partner, you have unlimited sex, you experience love, you no longer have to go to singles nights, you have stability, you get to commit and be committed to.

Con > you have less time with your other friends and family, you are restricted to one partner, you have to be committed, you have to compromise.

It is not as easy as it seems, is it? Even something as great as finding a new partner still has some cons. What about this one?

Event > you win ten million dollars in a lottery

Pro > you never have to work again, you can live an extravagant life, you can provide for friends and family if you choose to, you can buy expensive toys, you can live in an excellent home, you have no more financial worries.

Con > you will have all your friends and family coming to you asking for money, people will put pressure on how you spread your new wealth, people will seek donations, some friends may be jealous, you will feel pressure on what to do with the money, you might get bored, your kids might develop a cocaine addiction, your kids might be spoilt brats, you will now have to spend time managing this large amount of money, your expenses will most likely increase in line with your new wealth.

It is now clear that there is always a price to pay. What about something that seems like a negative event?

Event > you unexpectedly lose your job

Con > you need to find a new job urgently, you have no income, you have increased uncertainty, you may build up bad debt, you might have to adjust your lifestyle, you might have to change fields, you might not find a job.

Pro > you have new opportunities, you can try something new, you might find a better job, you might get an idea, you might change your lifestyle to something better, you might redesign your mind while you wait for a new job (see what I did there?).

These stories confirm that no matter what happens in life, there is always a pro and always a con. We can use this to cultivate thoughts of hope and understanding when the outcome does not go our way, and thoughts and feelings of gratitude and humbleness when the outcome is what we wanted. Whenever a negative thought-forming event occurs, write out the pros and cons and watch how your negative emotions are countered over time.

BE A MAGNET FOR POSITIVE ENERGY

The energy that you put out is what you attract. Positive, happy people attract other positive, happy people. It is as simple as that. And it doesn't mean that you have to be 100% positive 100% of the time but it means that your starting position is *positive*. If you were to think of yourself being in one of three gears; negative gear, neutral gear, or positive gear – we want to be driving most of the time in positive gear. Sure, there will be times where we drop into neutral or even into the negative, but it doesn't take us long to switch it back into positive gear to get moving forward again. I still get pissed off from time to time – I am still human and I want you to be too! We just have a redesigned mind.

Actively pursuing this positive energy and being a magnet for others has made a massive difference to my relationships and my own happiness. It sounds silly but people actually talk to you differently when you have a positive outlook. Even if you are calling a phone company to make a complaint, you would be surprised how you get treated differently if you are positive and understanding instead of negative and irritable. Do you smile whenever you get the chance? Even when you are addressing a checkout operator at a fast food joint; you would be amazed by how many free chicken nuggets you get if you just smile and be genuinely polite. Let me say it is not about the free chicken nuggets; it is about the feeling of gratitude, happiness and respect for yourself and others.

I don't know what it is but the energy you give out genuinely makes a difference to what happens to you in your day to day life. The sceptics will call me crazy, and that is ok because I know that it is just their mind putting up a defence as to why they don't need to be positive all the time. The best answer to this scepticism is actually a question. What are the costs of being positive? Whilst I don't have any hard evidence on this one, I don't think it uses much energy to smile. It doesn't cost you any money or any extra time to be genuinely positive and friendly to someone. So why not do it? Find your positive gear and stick to it as often as you can. It will go a long way to redesigning your mindset and helping your mind search for the positives in any situation.

FIND YOUR BEST FRIEND

Imagine you stuffed up something that was really important. A big exam, a relationship, a job interview, something you worked hard on. Whatever it is, how do you usually react? What do you say to yourself? Are you saying things such as 'you stuffed up', or 'you're an idiot', or 'you always screw things up', or 'you'll never find anyone' or 'you'll never be good enough', or my personal favourite, 'you're a loser'. In the previous chapters we looked at rewriting our thoughts which will definitely help change the tone of our language and remove these cognitive distortions, however we need to learn to *be our own best friend*.

Let's now imagine your best friend just broke up with her boyfriend. She has come around to your house for support and an evening away from the ex. Would you tell your best friend that she is a loser? Would you say that she will never find someone? Would you call her ugly? Would you say that she didn't try hard enough to make the relationship work? Of course not! You would put on Bridget Jones Diary (sorry ladies I only said this because I like this movie too), fill her with good vibes, talk her up and make her feel good about herself. You would be a rock for her. You can see where I am going with this, can't you?

So why would we help our friend during such a tough time, yet when it is our own lives and ourselves that we are talking to, we aren't so kind. Why are we quick to judge and criticise our actions? Why are we tearing ourselves down when we know exactly what we need to do to build ourselves up? It is time to scrap this self-debilitating mindset and develop our mind as our best friend. You are always there for yourself in good times and bad. You will always be there for all the highs, all the lows, and always do what you think is right for yourself. You put in all the effort for yourself. It is time now to love yourself just as you would your best friend. We are taught to treat others how we would like to be treated. Now it is time that we start treating *ourselves* in that same way.

REDESIGN YOUR MIND

CHAPTER FOURTEEN
YOU CAN CHANGE

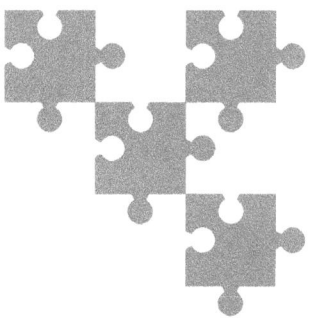

For those who have seen *The Wolf of Wall Street*, many of you will know that Jordan Belfort was a crook who ripped people off to get rich. At one point in time throughout Jordan's life he was a dick. But does this mean that he is labelled as a dick forever? Was there not a point when he was young, sweet and potentially *innocent*? If so that would mean that at some point in time he *changed*? Something must have happened for him to change into the person he became. After paying for his crimes in one way or another, he wrote a book and made a movie that brought a lot of enjoyment and taught many lessons to many people around the world. Could we now label him as something else? I mean he could have got out of jail and been ashamed of himself for the rest of his life, but instead he chose to embrace his story, hold himself accountable for his wrongdoings and tell his story to the world. Could we now say that he is now something special? One quote I love from the movie is, 'The only thing standing between you and your goal is the bullshit story you keep telling yourself as to why you can't achieve it'. Are we all guilty of this at times? I know I am. Redesigning your mind is something challenging and I am sure there are many reasons why you *shouldn't* have to do it. I know most of the excuses because I said them all myself. Now is the time where we stop making bullshit excuses. Now is the time where we acknowledge that it is going to be tough but we are going to do it anyway.

We are all fearful of change. It is how we are wired. Let's put that aside and face the fear with a new mindset. We have been changing and redesigning our minds and lives ever since we were born – we just haven't paid attention to it. Now is the time to embrace the never-ending redesign of our lives. I know that change can be scary but we need to remember that we can use our language and thoughts to empower us instead of hinder us. Change can be exciting. Change can be something new that we cannot wait to see. So much of our change is out of our control anyway; the economy, getting older, what is cool and what is not are all things that are going to change over time whether you like it or not. So you can choose to disregard it, dislike it, disagree with it, be disappointed by it, feel threatened by it; or you can choose to embrace it, want it and need it. Either way change is coming so you might as well actively pursue it and grab it with both hands.

One thing that I love about redesigning your mind is that there is absolutely nothing stopping you from being the person you want to be right now. You can literally change who you are just like that. You can literally go from being a senior legal executive to a part-time-barista who spends the other three days a week sitting on the beach. You have the power to sell all your stuff and get a one way ticket to India to find yourself. It's up to you. For too long we have put up these imaginary prison bars that force us to stay in the lives that once upon a time we thought were good for us. Why do we have to stick to something that we decided was right for us in the past but may not be right for us right now? Do you stick with a plan that no longer serves you or do you change your plan?

I hope that you have found some inspiration, some empowerment, some strength and some confidence to make any change that you want to make. You and only you live your life. There is no pause or rewind button, so you have to live it right the first time. If you feel that you are letting other people down, go back and rewrite your thoughts as to *why* you feel that way. Do you really think that these people that you are letting down really want you to be miserable with your life? I don't think so. They only want you to be happy.

You need to ask yourself if you want to actively make some changes in your life that are going to potentially bring you true happiness. There is no doubt that some of the changes you make might be the wrong ones in the short term, but this is ok. No redesign of anything is perfect the first time. Redesigning something is all about taking it apart and making it better. This takes thought, time and patience. You need to ask yourself if you are happier going on the same way or if you would rather make a change to find out. Are you scared of what other people will think? If you usually wear conservative clothing and all of a sudden turn up to a party wearing something outlandish, do you think that people will talk? Probably. Does it matter? No. Will you be happy that you are wearing what you want to wear? Of course! Have a laugh and have some fun with the redesign of your mind and your life.

It is amazing how much we can change within such a short time. Our perception of who we are and other people's perception of who they think we are can also change just as quickly. Looking back at my life so far I know that who I was and who I am now are totally different people. The funny thing is that I am still constantly redesigning and tweaking who I am. Just because you have been a certain person up until now it doesn't mean that you have to be that person tomorrow.

I know that things can seem dark and as if they will never recover at times but we have to remember that we still have the rest of our lives to find happiness. Take action now. If there is a girl/guy that you want to speak to, put this book down and send them a message. If she/he doesn't respond, then you know that no response *is* the response and you can move on. Find your meaning and use the reasons *why* you want to be who you want to be to light your fire of inspiration. I know you have it in you; otherwise you wouldn't have made it this far into the book! Start that hobby, act as if, redesign your mind, pick up that phone, join the sports team, sign up to the gym, leave work on time and throw out your old clothes. Whatever it is that you want to change – do it now; otherwise you will just waste your time thinking about it and risk never doing it all.

Think about yourself this time next week and how you will feel after making *any* change. How do you see yourself? You might still have a long way to go, but I guarantee that in a week there will be some *change* that you can feel good about. You might already look different or start to *feel* different. Compare this to yourself this time next week if you hadn't made *any* change. You might still be putting off your dreams. You might still be sitting next to someone that you don't want to. You might be working in a job that isn't right for you. You might still be in a toxic environment or cultivating toxic thoughts. You might not have taken any active step forward. How would you feel? Maybe you can't move a mountain by this time next week but you could carry away a few small stones. No one is pressuring you to redesign your mind or do anything else. This book is here to give you a few tools to help you on your journey if you want to take it. Ask yourself what you truly want and put a plan in place to make *some* progress by this time next week. I know you can do it. You just have to believe it yourself (*so cliché, Stef*).

Remember that the ultimate goal with change is happiness. It is great if you want to be more confident, or more charismatic, or be more active, or work less, or work more, or achieve a goal. Everything you want to do you do because you are seeking *happiness* from it. You don't want to be more confident just so that you can be more confident. You want to be more confident because having more confidence gives you the satisfaction that you *are confident*, which in turn makes you happy. All of these goals must tie into your happiness otherwise they will be wasting your time. As we talked about earlier, I used to think that money and a high social status would bring me happiness and hence why all my goals revolved around this. Now I know, as the research has proven, that large amounts of money and fame do not bring you happiness. I now believe this and my goals on life have totally changed. Redesigning my mind wasn't easy, and I still have fragments of the old mind which are constantly being worked on, but the great news is that I am more content with where I am in life than I have ever been before. Ready to face new challenges with a bag full of tools to help me on my way.

Your thoughts control your emotions and rewriting your thoughts is going to be a key part of your development. You can have all the support in the world but unfortunately until we can upload software to our brains like in the Matrix, you are going to have to do the hard work. To all of those people who have been on the edge of life and fear hitting this low again – it is ok. There is no need to fear the future because you only have to live today. Tomorrow doesn't exist yet. Working on your thoughts now and into the future will help you when times get tough. I have no doubt that as the good times come along, you can ease off on some of the practices in the book but know that they are here ready and waiting for you when you need them. If they don't work for you next time, try something else. Maybe there will be something new in the future. Never give up hope.

REDESIGNING CAN BE CHALLENGING

To acknowledge that something in your life is not right and that you have to redesign yourself is a challenge. Once you have accepted it, the redesign can actually be fun. You now get to decide what goes into your mind. Yes, it is a challenge to break habit and take yourself out of your comfort zone, but I can tell you that it will all be worth it. Yes, the fear that it won't work is something that you will have at the back of your mind but trust me when I say that it will help. Once you take that first step of a thousand miles, you will build your momentum and feel great when you look back at how far you have come. Do not get disheartened if things aren't moving too quickly at first and remember to keep building up the momentum. One step at a time. As your mind becomes aware of all the work that is needed it will try to convince you that it is all too hard. Tell yourself that it is only one step at a time that you need to focus on. Day by day you will get better and I can guarantee that the moment you have that initial, positive thought when you know you would have previously had a negative thought, you will be filled with confidence and joy!

Redesigning your mind will bring about challenges of your past. You will look back at your past with your new mindset and wonder how things could have turned out if you had this new mindset back then. This is nothing to be worried about and in fact it is a good thing. It means that you have learnt from this experience and you know you will tackle it differently with a new process next time. In my own life I sometimes wonder about the business that I closed, past friendships I had burnt and past relationships I had sabotaged. Sure, I could have made things work with my redesigned mindset, but it was not meant to be. This mindset was only created thanks to those experiences going the way they did. I am on a new path that is taking me to places I would never have gone with a mindset that I could never have imagined. I am grateful for where I am and do not waste any time on the 'what if' cognitive distortion. Life is not about looking at what could (or should) have been, life is about looking at where we are now and where we want to go. Whether it's a partner that we choose to stay with (or choose to leave), a lifestyle change, moving to another city – there will always be other paths we could have chosen.

Yes, we have to put in effort and we have to give things time to work, but I also want to challenge you and give you the confidence not to be scared to change paths. People might say that this is 'giving up' but I don't see it that way. I see it as actively deciding what you want to do. Staying in an environment or life that you don't want could be seen as 'giving up', so make sure you stay true to yourself and do not let others' opinions sway you either way. It is never too early, or never too late to change. Until we find that magical crystal ball that shows us exactly what we should do in each situation, there is no right answer. All you can do is write out your thoughts, fill in your journal and make the decision that seems right for you at the time.

21 DAYS OF CHANGE

Research shows it takes 21 days to make (or break) a habit. This is really a short amount of time. Can you commit yourself to 21 days of cultivating your new mindset in the hope of living a better life? Will you practice rewriting your thoughts morning and night for 21 days straight? I know you can! No longer will you make excuses as to why you 'can't do something' and instead you will talk about how good it feels to be responsible for cultivating your own mindset. Take each day as one small step on your journey of a thousand miles.

Please remember that you don't have to stick to the same changes for the rest of your life. Redesigning your mind is all about constant re-evaluation and self-development. What works for you at this moment might not work in the future. That is totally cool; keep changing and redesign yourself again and again. Life is always evolving and new challenges will always present themselves. We need to keep evolving too. Our mindset, attitude, health, fitness and the way we live our lives always need to keep changing with the times. If Austin Powers taught us anything it is that you need to evolve with the times or be left behind. You are groovy baby and I know you can redesign your life just as I have.

CHAPTER FIFTEEN
A LIFE OF REDESIGN

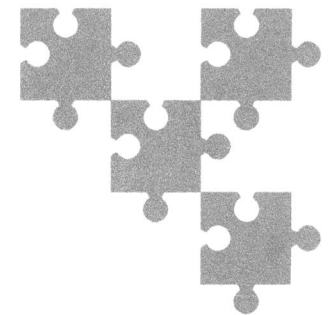

REDESIGN COMPLETE...FOR NOW

I hope that I am leaving you with a new-found passion for wellness. I hope you have discovered a passion to constantly evolve, to constantly seek new ways to better yourself and to improve your happiness. Redesign your mind does not mean that you change and then that is it. It means that we *redesign* the way we think about change and acknowledge that we will never stop. Throughout my life I have always wanted things wrapped up into a neat little package so that I can move on to the next thing. Whenever I wanted to change something in my life I would hope that it wouldn't take long and would expect results pretty quickly. I learnt that this is not how you cultivate a positive mindset. A positive mindset takes time, and just like a well-manicured garden it requires time, care and maintenance to stay beautiful. Appreciate and enjoy the journey of redesigning your mind because once you're happy with the change and the way your life is, new challenges will present themselves.

You will screw up at some stage and that is ok. Accept that you will remain human and you will make mistakes. As discussed earlier, *Thinking, Fast and Slow* by Daniel Kahneman mentions that as humans we tend to look back in hindsight as if a decision that we got wrong, *should* have been easy to get right. No longer will we criticize ourselves for something that we weren't expected to know. The more you screw up the better you will get at it. The more you laugh at yourself and not punish yourself for not keeping your perfect record the happier you will be. I now take responsibility for my stuff ups instead of using 'The Blamer' cognitive distortion. I now use 'process v outcome' to determine whether or not I can learn something from a negative outcome, instead of using the 'Labelling' cognitive distortion and calling myself a loser. I now ask myself 'does it really matter?' instead of using the 'magnification' cognitive distortion and blowing up a small problem. Sure, my mind still flicks back to negative thoughts regularly, but when it does I write down my thoughts and work through them – instead of ruminating on the same negative thought over and over, leading to an anxiety attack or a depressive state.

Every day I choose to be grateful for what I have got. I work harder than I ever have towards my goals, seeking to fulfil my meaning – but I don't hold back my happiness, waiting until life is complete before I can be happy. Otherwise I won't be happy until I am on my death bed! Speaking of death beds, yesterday approximately 150,000 people died and left this world for good. As you are reading this book you are 'luckier' than most of those people who would give anything to see another day of life. There is already something to be grateful for. Life itself. Do you want to have to wait until you are on your death bed before you become grateful for the experiences that you have had; the good times, the challenges, your friends and your family? Or do you want to be grateful for those things now and smile and acknowledge how amazing your life actually is? You know that being grateful is going to make you a happier person so why not stop and smell the roses?

Each and every day we have to choose what thoughts we are going to empower and what thoughts we are going to let float by. This ultimately will affect how you feel and whether emotions of anxiety and depression or joy and gratitude present themselves. Regardless of your positive attitude and new mindset, you need to be clear on your goals. Your meaning. Your purpose. Your reason for being here. Like me, you might find that some of the goals you had in the past are actually *fake* goals that are just wasting your time. For me, money and validation from the outside world was something I previously longed and strived for. Not that I ever became 'rich' but I did have a fair amount of money as a young person– yet I wasn't happy and I just wanted more. As I slipped further and further away from a balanced life, I realised that what I could achieve with my successful career and riches was not going to bring me half as much happiness as my family and friends would. Using the excuse that I needed heaps of money to help fund my family goals was also proven to be a load of shit as soon as the research showed me that money truly doesn't buy happiness. We need to spend time 'sitting on the balcony' looking down at ourselves, reviewing our lives and what else we may need to change. Ask yourself how you are going? Are you on the right path? How did you handle yourself this week? We need to actively dedicate time to our own development as a human being. Before reading this book, when was the last time you sat down for a day and planned out your life, your goals, your meaning and your mindset? Maybe you are like me and never sat down to actively work on all of those things as a whole. Now is the time to take ourselves to the mind-gym and get those mind-muscles moving. You have all the tools to help you and a new awareness and inspiration to keep you going when times get tough. Don't be scared to engage a psychologist (personal trainer for the mind) to help you on your journey. You will never know until you give it a go!

SHIT TIMES WILL COME AND GO

Even though I have redesigned my mind, it doesn't mean that I don't have shit times. I face all the same challenges I used to face and I can still feel anxious or depressed at times. The difference is that now I have a meaning, the right tools and a positive mindset to help me get through the shit times. 'Bad' things may happen again in the future but it is up to me to decide how I am going to react and move forward. No longer will I be jealous of the person who has it easier than I did. No longer will I be disappointed when the outcome doesn't turn out the way I want. I now take responsibility for my actions and for my feelings. I choose the thoughts that replay in my mind and I choose how I am going to spend my day.

These will be challenges that we need to be brave for. These shit times are things we need to accept and understand. We need to endure them to enjoy the good times. Mike Tyson said that 'everyone has a plan until they get punched in the face'. I love this quote. How can we expect to go through the boxing match of life without getting punched in the face every now and then? By having the right mental framework and tools ready to help us when the punch in the face comes we will be better able to deal with it. Don't worry, my book will always be waiting for you whenever you need it most. *We cannot stop the waves but we can learn to surf.* Just like the story where we journey towards our own paradise beach; there are always going to be challenges to face before you get to anywhere special.

What shit times have you experienced in your life that have given you an excuse to give up? Have you become envious because someone you know has had success and you haven't; or angry because they haven't had to face the same challenges as you? We need to learn to accept that this is the way it is and start doing something to improve our outlook on life. We can take responsibility for our actions and be happy for anyone else who has success. The alternative is to complain or give up and accept that you have been defeated (by yourself). I hope this helps you when times get tough. Just like the rest of this book, I expect to read this out to myself when things get tough to help remember that shit times will come and shit times will go. Just like my story of paradise beach, you will find that every challenge and every hurt is always forgotten when you experience just one moment of pure happiness.

WHERE AM I NOW

You might think that I now spend most of my days practicing yoga, eating acai bowls, sitting on the beach, meditating and writing out my thoughts – well that's what my family and friends joke about anyway. Whilst this would be a pretty awesome way to spend most of my time, I am now fairly busy with a much more balanced lifestyle. I still work full time in finance while maintaining a balanced lifestyle that brings me much joy. Redesigning my mind hasn't taken away any of my motivation or drive for success – it has just *redefined* what I mean by success. Now I am working towards *real* goals and also work hard at achieving a *balanced* lifestyle. Working hard is not just about work these days – it is about making time for family, friends, fitness, mental health, relationships and having fun. My blog 'The Wellness of Health' helps me spread the word on the importance of mental health. I guess I could say that I am now a bit of a wellness junkie – but that's a label that I wouldn't call a cognitive distortion.

It was around three years ago that I decided to redesign my mind and my life for the better. It started by figuring out what was *really* important to me and then changing both my mindset and my environment to suit. I have challenged myself to do things that are out of my comfort zone and pushed myself to do things differently. I have questioned who I was and why I wanted to be that person. Now I have *redefined* who I am and I am happy with this – for now. I'm not any more special than anyone else but I am living a much better life – and that is what redesigning your mind is all about. Things can *change* so quickly which is one of the greatest things about life. Yes, I still get anxious, disappointed and even depressed – but what has changed is how I react to these feelings. How I work through these challenging emotions has given me back the control. That said, I do know that things can change quickly. For this reason I do not take my happiness for granted and every day I accept that tomorrow my life could *change* for better or worse. But I accept that no matter what the *outcome* is, I can always ask myself whether I had the right *processes* or not. If something went wrong on my part, well then I have learnt to accept responsibility and cop it on the chin. No longer will I use the 'entitled brat' cognitive distortion and expect that my life *should* be better than anyone else's.

I now try my best not to think about the stresses of today or what stresses are on the agenda for tomorrow. I know all too well that the little dramas in life are what can keep you down and not enjoying the moment. Something as small as my sports team losing a football match would previously have somewhat depressed the rest of my weekend. Now I have a laugh about it. Why would I be depressed? I was only on the sidelines watching. I still support them and there is always next week. There were still some positives in the game, like that awesome goal in the third quarter or that hanger of a mark my favourite player took in the first. What thoughts you focus on will ultimately drive your emotions. Fuel your energy by staying in positive gear as often as possible and watch how far you can go.

After that holiday to the USA which kick-started my emotions of anxiety and depression, boarding a plane to Europe after I redesigned my mind, all on my own did bring about some challenging thoughts. *Would I get sick again? Would I get depressed? Would I be a loser? Would I not have a good time over here? Would everyone think I was a loser when I got back home with nothing exciting to say?* Yeah, they were floating around my head, but I knew how to deal with them. By rewriting my thoughts and using the tools in this book, I went to Europe and had the time of my life. This trip rekindled my love for travel and new experiences. If I hadn't redesigned my mind and faced those challenges, maybe I never would have left little old Adelaide for a holiday again. I am most grateful that I made the decision to commit to myself and hold myself accountable.

There is going to be the day that whatever you are doing right now, you will not be able to do anymore. If you are holding your baby in your arms, there will come a day when your baby will turn into an adult. If you enjoy travelling the world, one day you will be too old to climb the steps of the Great Wall of China. If you enjoy painting, playing sport, playing an instrument, or climbing a mountain, one day your body will not physically be able to do it. If you have something in your head that you want to do, and it is possible to do, then go and do it right now. Nothing will be worse than lying on your death bed when it is all too late contemplating what could have been. You do not want to be wishing you tried something, wishing you were a nicer person, or wishing you had chance to go back and make up with a special person in your life. Now is the time to set an agenda for the rest of your life and get to work on making it all happen. The only way to guarantee that you give it your all is to start today.

I know that I still have room for improvement on my journey of self-development. That is really the best part. Knowing that I have come so far and yet I can still do so much more leaves me feeling excited for the future. I am happy to keep changing and evolving by taking on new experiences. When redesigning your mind, it is important not to pressure yourself to 'get better fast' or to do anything you are not capable of doing yet. Start small. Remember you can move mountains just by starting to move a few small stones.

THE MENTAL HEALTH STIGMA

During the first phases of my recovery, I started a job as a financial planner. One of the first things I did was apply for life insurance and income protection – because a large part of financial planning is recommending life insurance and this was something I didn't have in place for myself yet. When I was going through the process I knew that there would be an 'exclusion' for mental health due to my recent battles with anxiety and depression. Oh, and by the way, an exclusion is where an insurer says that they will insure you for your life excluding particular events – in my case I was expecting the insurer to exclude mental health events (e.g. suicide or acts of harm to myself). I received a call from my financial planner (who was also a work colleague) saying that he had some bad news in that the insurer didn't want to give me any insurance. He recommended that I withdraw my application before it was declined. *What me? Nothing? Why not?* I was a young, fit, healthy person with no medical history other than having my recent challenge with mental health, and they didn't want to insure me. Yes, I had headaches and symptoms of numerous ailments however after testing everything possible the doctors declared again and again that it was all in my head and that there was nothing wrong with me. Yet my own employer said that I was too risky to insure so I withdrew my application. Besides the embarrassment of having my colleague know that I had all these challenges in the past, and the fear that he could tell everyone about it, it was the fact that I was too much of a risk to an insurer that hurt the most. How was I going to recommend life insurances to clients when I had nothing in place for myself? This was just another hurdle to overcome.

I could have let this defeat me. I could have let this be an embarrassing stain on my record, but instead I chose to embrace it. I wrote my thoughts out and looked for the *pros* of this *con*. I found the positives and moved on stronger than ever. I embraced the fact that I was probably one of the few financial planners in Australia without life insurance. I would actively tell clients that I wished I was in their chair and had the opportunity to put insurance in place. I explained the risks of not getting cover today may mean that you cannot get it in the future, at a time when you really need it. I explained that because of my mental health issues in the past, I am unable to put insurances in place which meant that I was unprotected. Clients really appreciated this and understood the importance of getting the right protection when they can – because like anything in life you never know when things can change. I learnt that by embracing my past and looking at the positives, not only were my emotions much better, but my energy and enthusiasm towards the topic turned it into a moment of strength instead of a moment of weakness.

Believe it or not there are many people just like you and me who have seen psychologists, or have had brain fog, or are stressed out, or have had breakdowns. For me, this was one thing that really helped me get over the fact that I was 'uninsurable' at the time. I went from feeling like an outcast to realising that there are many other people just like us. It is time for us to raise awareness and help others understand that people do not need to feel like an outcast when they are diagnosed with anxiety or depression. We are the ones who are 'normal'. You can sit with the rest of us who are conscientious, self-aware, and who totally give a f*ck about themselves and the people around them. You are alive and once you *change* you are going to feel emotions of happiness far greater than those who haven't embraced their emotions. We need to help those who think that anyone with a mental illness is 'weak' because they are a hazard to themselves and those around them. Their negative energy and thoughts towards anxiety and depression will not allow them to fully support those who are going through it – and will leave them feeling ashamed and embarrassed if it ever happens to them. We need to embrace the ignorant and not send anger towards them. Together we will redesign the importance of mental health and how the world sees it.

We aren't going to stop many of the negative events in life but we can *change* how we react to them. We can also redesign how we see our day to day lives. Dealing with mental illness is a part of life that every person on this planet is going to face at some point in their lives – whether they know it or not. Whether it is they themselves who face it or someone they know – it will happen. We need to accept these challenges and make mental health a part of normal life and conversation. We cannot dwell on the fact that someone is depressed or had a break down. We need to embrace these challenges and help everyone understand that it is ok not to be ok. It is time to work together on changing the world and making mental health cool – just like losing weight or having a makeover. We need to start looking at mental health experts and dealing with mental health just like any other activity to fix or improve your life. They are our personal trainers for the mind and seeing one is nothing we should be worried or ashamed about. We need to make mental health so popular that they turn it into a reality show like *The Biggest Loser*. Maybe there could be a mental health version of *The Biggest Loser*? *Reverse pun intended – laugh a little bit!*

We all need to embrace our mental health and continue to work on it. Continue to learn, continue to redesign and continue to strive to be the happiest person you can be. And now we all know that monetary or material success is not what we are looking for, we can focus on meaningful goals. Sustained, long term happiness based on love and gratitude is what we are after. Think about what you can do to help remove the mental health stigma. I don't have all the answers but I do know that we need, as a society, to redesign how we see mental health – because even in this connected fast-paced world we live in, you can be cold and lonely when you are depressed or anxious. We need to create a world where anxiety and depression are just states of emotion that we can change through our actions and thoughts; and not allow these emotions to remain as beasts lurking in the shadows that can rule our life. Help make the change and join me by redesigning yourself first.

OVER TO YOU

Well it is now the part of the book where I say goodbye and its over to you to get to work. I have shown you some of the challenges that I have faced and how I redesigned my mind. My life is far from perfect; and just today I got angry for something trivial. But within a few minutes I was having a laugh at myself and realised that it was something that I wouldn't care about in a few days – so why care about it now? I am leaving you with a bag full of tools to help you redesign your mind and get you from where you are now to where you want to be. I hope that these tools and the inspiration of my story have helped you to level up your mental health.

CHAPTER FIFTEEN – A LIFE OF REDESIGN

The thing about my life now is that I have no idea which way it is going to go – which I am happy about for once. I am still only 30 years old but it feels like a lifetime away since I faced my battle with mental illness in my early to mid 20's. I truly did struggle with understanding and respecting my emotions and I was trying to live up to an image that society created for me. Not saying that I am smart, but for a person who has a fast-thinking mind, dealing with anxiety and depression was something that my 'entitled brat' cognitive distortion thought I didn't need to face. This made it much worse in the short term, but in the long term it has enabled me to learn so much and even to write a book that will hopefully help so many people.

I urge you to make a new start upon finishing this book. Draw a line in the sand right here and now and say that this is the moment that you can start to redesign your mind and decide to walk the path that you lay out for yourself. The changes that you make today are going to give you the greatest chance of living your happiest life. It is time to forget about what someone else's visions of happiness and success are and make your own version. Find your meaning of life and create a life that fulfils this meaning.

Love for others and most importantly love for yourself is something that you must always cultivate. Remember that change is going to have its ups and downs and learn to cut yourself some slack. Treat yourself like you would your best friend because you will always be there for yourself no matter what happens. Now is the time to reshape who you are. Remember that there is absolutely nothing stopping you from totally reinventing yourself – now and again in the future. No one is and can ever hold you back from redesigning your mind and redesigning your life. You can throw out your clothes and create a new look for yourself within minutes – why not do the same for your personality? You can *change* anything that you like. You just have to give yourself the power. I am sure that this book has inspired you to redesign your mind, but if it hasn't, or if you lose the inspiration somewhere along the way, does that mean that you can now give up? Does that mean that you can accept that this is your life and that there is nothing you can do about it? Or can you find a way to acknowledge this book as something that has helped you on your journey? Acknowledge that there is still a world full of experiences and tools that may help you improve your mental health in another way? Persistence will pay off. Finding your meaning will provide the inspiration you need to fuel your persistence. Belief will drive your persistence when you cannot see the light and could have easily given up. Believe in yourself and believe that you will level up your mental health and improve your happiness.

For those that aren't anxious or depressed and are just seeking more positivity or happiness – I applaud you for committing to such a task. You are an inspiration for those who want to improve themselves and take part in the pursuit of wellness. You may already have many of the tools and behaviours ingrained in your mind, but I am sure there are a few cognitive distortions that you can work on to get yourself to the next level. Maybe you are like a knight in shining armour who is here to help those who lack the skills and mindset that you are so blessed with. Take this as a calling and an opportunity to spread the word of your story and help those who are less fortunate.

My story is just a snippet of what someone may go through. I hope it helps you realise that you can change and you will change if you give it time. We must accept the challenges but we must not accept that mental health is purely something out of our control, up to our genetics, or up to luck. We must acknowledge that we are responsible for the state of our mental health and no matter what our circumstances are, we can always improve.

Flashing back to when I was at the bottom of the barrel, on a beach with my dad when it was all too much for us to bare, I can tell you that moving from this beach of sadness, to my paradise beach, on a journey of change and self-development has been the best thing that I have ever done. Sitting there without the headaches, the tension, the dissociation and brain fog, or the pressure that I put on myself; well I guess that has made the journey of growth even more special. Who knows what the next chapter of my life will bring, but one thing I do know is that I face life with a redesigned mindset. I have levelled up and I am ready to face the new challenges with a bag full of tools to help me get through it. The question you need to ask yourself is what changes are you going to make and when will you make them? Right now? Tomorrow? Next week when things aren't so busy? We both know the answer as to when the right time is. As for what to change, well I guess that will be up to you.

The best part about redesigning your mind is that you can do it again and again. What may be a perfectly redesigned mind for you today may not be the mind that works for you tomorrow. Life is about constant change. This constant change will mean that your mindset will need to change too. Yes, you may have a new positively set foundation that will never need to move – but you will need to update the contents of *what really matters* as time goes on. Ultimately the ones that continuously pursue the redesign of their minds will be the ones that live the most fulfilled lives – well that's what I think anyway. Even though I wrote this book that I hope will help so many people, I know that I too will have to find new ways to redesign my mind in the future. The good news is that now I understand how empowering this can be and I look forward to creating the new best version of me. It is now up to you to decide if you will join me.

THE CHECKLIST TO REDESIGN YOUR MIND

Wow, you have come a long way on the journey to redesigning your mind. It is amazing to look back and see all the tools, practices and behaviours that you have learned about in this book. Some of you might only need to tick off a few things while some of the perfectionist wankers like me will try and tick them all off. Either way my advice is not to use this checklist as something to get through quickly. I was going to write down how many times you 'should' do each item before you can tick it off, but I will leave that up to you. The redesigning of your mind is a constant work in progress. Even after you have ticked something off you can decide to do it again. Feel free to share on social media what worked, what didn't work and what you added to your own list to redesign your mind.

CHECKLIST TO REDESIGN YOUR MIND
☐ Know and understand the cognitive distortions and which ones are most prevalent in you
☐ Practice rewriting your thoughts 5 days out of 7 (at least 15 minutes morning and night)
☐ Figure out and write down your own meaning of life
☐ Write out the Pros v Cons for a particular negative situation
☐ Contact your GP / Medical Practitioner for a physical health and mental health assessment
☐ Engage a psychologist (personal trainer for the mind)
☐ Change at least one thing in your environment
☐ Practice the 'Process v Outcome' tool
☐ Practice the '5-minute summary of the day' with at least one person
☐ Incorporate 'Act as If' into your mind
☐ Spread the word of your progress using #redesignyourmind on social media
☐ Give this book to someone else – or even better tell them to buy their own copy!
☐ Forgive someone who wronged you. Apologise to them for any wrongdoing on your part
☐ Go two weeks without saying the word 'should'

☐	Work out the areas that are important to you and how much time and energy you want to spend in each of these areas
☐	Do something that scares you
☐	Say sorry to someone you wronged in your past
☐	Write out a journal. Specifically, 'The Weekly Journal'
☐	Tell someone you love them (someone that you haven't said this to in recent times)
☐	Do something that you always wanted to do but never have done (or haven't for a long time)
☐	Redefine what social media does for you and be more observant of your actions
☐	Redefine what money means to you
☐	Redefine what success means to you
☐	Breathe. Put a prompt in place to remind yourself to breathe.
☐	Set up an exercise schedule for at least 30 minutes per session
☐	Decide on and write down what you actually give a f*ck about in life
☐	Practice Yoga
☐	Become your best friend. Talk to yourself as you would do to your best friend.
☐	Practice meditation
☐	Practice mindfulness
☐	Remove your expectations on something or someone
☐	Create a balanced diet for yourself. Start with 5 days of good and 2 days of treating yourself. Engage a nutritionist or dietician for professional help.
☐	Engage a positive mindset coach (you can engage me as your mindset coach at wellnessofhealth.com)
☐	Ask yourself 'does it really matter' to something that would have previously brought on negative thoughts and emotions
☐	Spread the word of mental illness and the importance of positive mental health
☐	Give someone a go – either in a friendship, relationship or in a situation where you would usually write them off before giving them a chance
☐	Give the placebo effect a chance – specifically for something that your old mindset would have written off before giving it a chance

STAY IN CONTACT

Redesign your mind is all about the journey of self-development. Together we can help end the mental health stigma and help people become the people that they want to be. Share the progress of your journey on social media by using the hash tag #redesignyourmind and tagging my Instagram account @wellnesshealth17.

Please feel free to get in contact with me. You can share your own story of how you redesigned your mind, ask questions, or even share new ways of how to take on the challenges of mental illness. I would love to hear from you. I also have a positive mindset coach program on my website if you are interested.

Website: www.wellnessofhealth.com

Insta: @Wellnesshealth17

YouTube: Wellness of Health

Facebook: Facebook.com/wellnessofhealth

ACKNOWLEDGEMENTS

If redesigning my mind was the hardest thing I have ever done, writing a book about it must be the next closest thing. Writing this book has been a massive test of how important wellness and mental health is to me. Just like you on your journey to redesign your mind, there have been times when I wanted to give up. At times the only thing that has kept me going is the thought that one day you will get to read it. The thought that you might get to benefit from this book pushed me to keep going. The amount of time, money, energy, blood, sweat and tears that I have put into making this book has been challenging but so worth it. The good news is that I haven't been the only one pushing to make this book into what it is. It is now time to thank those people who have helped in any way. Many of them deserve thanks without knowing it.

First of all thank you so much to my family. Without their sacrifices and hard work, I never would have had the opportunity to strive for my goals, fall down, learn and then build myself back up. During these tough times and dark days it was you that held me up and kept me moving forward. Without your love and support during the tough times who knows if I would have had the love and determination to redesign my mind and then write a book about it. I love you all and thank you dearly. To my friends; I love how you keep me grounded and love to take the piss out of me when I get too serious about my wellness journey and passion for improving everything imaginable. I wouldn't choose anyone else to enjoy life's journey with and I thank you so much for being there during the good times and bad. Thank you to my psychologist (personal trainer for the mind). Even though I only saw you for a handful of sessions, your guidance and wisdom sparked the inspiration in me to get me started on the redesign of my mind. Without your help I would never have had the tools to get started on this journey.

Thank you to my writing trainer and structural editor, Jennifer Althaus from Orange Elephants Creative Minds. I am forever grateful for finding you and taking on this journey with you. This book would not be half as good as it is without your insight, tough love and guidance. I thank you so much for taking on my project. Thank you to Leone Sperling for your grammar editing eye and for polishing this manuscript into a fine piece of art. Thanks to Evan Shapiro from Cilento Publishing. Your creativity and guidance on the finishing touches and cover design have helped deliver my message with such punch that I know many people will understand exactly what it means to redesign your mind.

Thank you to those that haven't been nice to me or have challenged me in some way over the years. Even though I didn't like it at the time, I know that your role in my life is as great as anyone's and I thank you for making me stronger, more understanding and grateful for the good times. You helped me level up. I also want to thank all of the people that have followed me and joined the journey on the Wellness of Health Blog along the way. Your collaboration and continuous support have been inspirational to me. I look forward to sharing the journey with you.

Thank you to each and every person who is helping to make a difference to people's mental health. Whether it is raising awareness, helping those in need or just being a good person – your efforts are having an impact on society and helping to remove the stigma around mental health. We have come so far as a society over the last few years, but I know that we still have a long way to go. Keep raising awareness, keep fighting, and keep sharing your story. You never know who you might be helping.

Finally, I want to thank you, the reader. You are the person that has chosen to read my story and put your time and faith into the tools that I think will help you with your mental health. Words can't describe how special it feels to know that you read so many of my pages! I hope that you enjoyed my story and learned something that will help you on your journey. Please feel free to share with me how you are going on your journey as I look forward to sharing more of your stories on how you redesigned your mind on my blog and hopefully my next book. Thank you so much.

REFERENCES

Beyondblue.org.au. (2019). Beyond Blue. [online] Available at: https://www.beyondblue.org.au/about-us/research-projects/statistics-and-references [Accessed 2 Feb. 2019].

Cdc.gov. (2017). Products - Data Briefs - Number 283 - August 2017. [online] Available at: https://www.cdc.gov/nchs/products/databriefs/db283.htm [Accessed 2 Feb. 2019].In page citation

Dorey, F. (2018). *Homo sapiens – modern humans.* [online] The Australian Museum. Available at: https://australianmuseum.net.au/learn/science/human-evolution/homo-sapiens-modern-humans/ [Accessed 13 Feb. 2019].

Burns, D. (1980). *Feeling Good: The New Mood Therapy.* William Morrow and Company Inc., pp.14-15.

Blackdoginstitute.org.au. (2019). One hour of exercise a week can prevent depression. [online] Available at: https://blackdoginstitute.org.au/news/news-detail/2017/10/04/one-hour-of-exercise-a-week-can-prevent-depression [Accessed 24 Feb. 2019].

Abs.gov.au. (2019). 3303.0 - Causes of Death, Australia, 2017. [online] Available at: https://www.abs.gov.au/ausstats/abs@.nsf/Lookup/by%20Subject/3303.0~2017~Main%20Features~Intentional%20self-harm,%20key%20characteristics~3 [Accessed 24 Feb. 2019].

Ducharme, J. (2018). *This Is the Amount of Money You Need to Be Happy, According to Research* [online] Money.com. Available at: http://money.com/money/5157625/ideal-income-study/ [Accessed 14 Apr. 2019].

Yutang, L. (1998). *The Importance of Living.* p.159.

RECOMMENDED READING

Feeling Good: The New Mood Therapy (1980) by David Burns

This book is jam packed with tools and strategies to help overcome anxiety and depression. This is the book most responsible for giving me the tools and belief to change my life. You won't need to use all the tools in the book, but this could be your new bag of tools for feeling good.

The Worry Cure (2005) by Robert Leahy

You might find this similar to *Feeling Good*, however it is more aimed at anxiety and worry. For someone like me, a lot of my depression started from worry and this book does a great job of helping you rationalise those fears. It even builds on some of the tools from *Feeling Good*.

Thinking Fast and Slow (2011) by Daniel Kahneman

This book is for those that want a fact filled, heavy read on how the mind works. It doesn't really focus on tools to help you change, but it is more about understanding that our mind can be influenced. This is a book that requires a lot of heavy, numbers style thinking – so make sure it appeals to you before you pick it up and dedicate some time to it.

Mastering your Hidden Self: A Guide to the Huna Way (A Quest Book) (1985) by Serge Kahili King

This is a great read about cultures which are different to our Western World. It demonstrates that a lot of our anxiety and depression may be caused by our own thoughts, which we can be freed from. I like this because it helped me understand that our environment and thought processes are what influence how we feel. More for those on the spiritual side.

*The Subtle Art of Not Giving a F*ck* (2016) by Mark Manson

I have a love hate relationship with this book, but it is still a great read. If you feel that you give a f*ck too much, then this book is for you. It is an easy, light hearted read that will give you a few laughs and help you understand that you don't need to give a f*ck about things that aren't important to you. The book works well in conjunction with some of the more theoretical and technical books above.

A New Earth: Awakening Your Life's Purpose (2005) by Eckhart Tolle

You may have heard of Tolle's other book, *The Power of Now* (1997) – which was extremely popular and well recommended by none other than Oprah. *The Power of Now* is a little more on the spiritual side, and whilst it helped me a great deal with my challenges, I found that *A New Earth* is more practical and gives you more of an understanding of one of our flaws as humans – our ego. Some of us that may be egotistic or striving too hard for our goals could really benefit from reading this book.

Man's Search for Meaning (1946) by Viktor E Frankl

This book tells the true story of a Jewish psychologist being held in a Nazi concentration camp during World War II. His findings on how we can use our 'meaning' or purpose to get through unthinkable challenges is something that is really inspiring.

Sapiens, A Brief History of Humankind (2011) by Yuval Noah Harari

This is a great read for those that want to learn more about the evolution humankind and how we as Homo sapiens came to rule the world. Thought provoking and will lead you into questioning whether we need much of the luxuries that we seek in today's world.

www.ingramcontent.com/pod-product-compliance
Lightning Source LLC
Chambersburg PA
CBHW051947290426
44110CB00015B/2139